HEALTH OPTIONS

Andrew Vickers researches and writes about complementary medicine. He currently works for the Research Council for Complementary Medicine, which promotes scientific research in the complementary therapies. He has also had experience of working with disabled people in the community.

Health Options

COMPLEMENTARY THERAPIES
FOR CEREBRAL PALSY
AND RELATED CONDITIONS

Andrew Vickers
Research Council for Complementary Medicine

Published in association with
The Spastics Society

ELEMENT
Shaftesbury, Dorset ● Rockport, Massachusetts
Brisbane, Queensland

First published in Great Britain in 1994 by
Element Books Ltd
Shaftesbury, Dorset

Published in the USA in 1994 by
Element, Inc.
42 Broadway, Rockport, MA 01966

Published in Australia in 1994 by
Element Books Ltd
for Jacaranda Wiley Ltd
33 Park Road, Milton, Brisbane, 4064

Cover design by Max Fairbrother
Design by Roger Lightfoot
Typeset by Footnote, Warminster, Wiltshire
Printed and bound in Great Britain by
Redwood Books Ltd, Trowbridge, Wiltshire

British Library Cataloguing in Publication
data available

Library of Congress Cataloging in Publication
data available

ISBN 1-85230-562-2

The production of this publication has been made possible by the generous support of Lloyds Bank, as part of its ongoing community programme.

The Spastics Society is the largest charity in the country working with people with cerebral palsy, their parents and carers.

The Spastics Society (to be named SCOPE from November 1994) believes there will be a number of ways in which the physical tensions experienced by people with cerebral palsy can be eased. No one way will be of benefit to all people.

We welcome this book and its exploration of additional therapy options which may complement existing methods and extend choice to people with cerebral palsy, their parents and carers.

Contents

Foreword

In recent years, I have enjoyed the benefits of some complementary therapies in conjunction with traditional medicine, and have often wished the benefits I was enjoying could be extended to people with disabilities. During this time, we in the Spastics Society/SCOPE carried out some preliminary work and found a great need for further investigation.

Physiotherapy, which is somewhat limited during school-days, becomes more of a rarity later on. It would seem to me that the prescribing of painkilling drugs is far too often the only available solution to alleviate discomfort of any sort.

As a parent of a young woman born with cerebral palsy I have always known not to look for a cure. When Ann was young, my wish was always for more improvement physically, and to maintain good health. However, to quote my daughter, now aged 37, 'Mum, cerebral palsy marches on!', obviously bringing with it some deterioration of unused muscles and limbs.

For younger and older people with disabilities, therefore, the best quality of life in the situation in which they find themselves, must always be a major objective. Housing, and a sympathetic environment which caters for everyday needs and incentives are important, but equally important is the opportunity to achieve a feeling of peace with one's own body and disability, and to live as comfortably as possible.

The one-to-one relationship provided by a qualified practitioner of complementary therapies, sensitive to the needs of disabled people is invaluable. Even a simple massage is relaxing, helping general circulation and muscle tone, and there are, as this book describes, a wide range of other therapies.

I am convinced that some complementary therapies bring cumulative benefits and comfort to people with disabilities, offering them at least a partial alternative to the obvious prescribing of drugs. My hope is that the medical profession's cautious interest and involvement in complementary therapies will grow, and that they will work towards providing facilities for more of this important work to be carried out.

I am delighted that it has been possible to produce this book written so ably by Andrew Vickers, and I would like to thank Jim Hoskisson and Raficq Abdulla of The Spastics Society/SCOPE who have supported the concept from the beginning and encouraged it through its various stages.

Eileen Milnes
Former Vice-Chairman
The Spastics Society

Preface

The aim of this book is to allow people affected by cerebral palsy and related conditions to make informed decisions about their health options. Unbiased information on complementary therapies has always been difficult to obtain. Most orthodox health professionals have little training in or knowledge of complementary medicine and are therefore often unable to give suitable advice. Books and leaflets on complementary medicine are generally written by practitioners and rarely have the necessary degree of objectivity. Moreover, though many people hear about complementary therapies from friends, it is difficult to come to any useful conclusions about a therapy based on just one friend's or colleague's experience.

The author of this book is a professional writer and researcher in complementary medicine. He has never been a health practitioner and therefore has no axe to grind. He was chosen by The Spastics Society specifically because of this objectivity and because of his experience in disability work.

Though this book focuses on cerebral palsy, it also makes reference to a variety of other neurodevelopmental disabilities. This book will be of interest to anyone who has or anyone who cares for someone who has a condition that stems from damage to or improper functioning of the nervous system at an early stage of life. Such conditions include Down's syndrome, tuberous sclerosis and many of the learning disabilities. Though the emphasis of the book is on the treatment of children, it should remain of interest to many adults with disabilities.

How to Read Health Options

This book had two main themes.

1. There are no quick or simple answers to complex health problems.
2. Healthcare should be approached in a systematic and organized way.

You should bear these two points in mind when you read this book. For example, it is not a good idea to flick through the index looking for quick information about particular therapies and health problems. To do so would be to miss much of the important background information of the first three chapters. Without this background, much of the rest of the book becomes meaningless or misleading. It is strongly recommended that you read all of Chapters 1, 2, 3 and 5. Chapter 4, however, describes a number of different therapies and you may feel that you only wish to read about those that interest you.

You may also like to consider – now, before you start reading – how you should read. Would it be best to read the whole book through in one go? Or to read twenty pages a day? Would it help if you took notes as you went along? What sort of information are you looking for? Reading this book in a systematic and organized way will help you achieve the aim of making an informed decision about complementary medicine.

How was the Information for This Book Gathered?

One of the best ways of gathering information about a therapy is to conduct a scientific trial. The problem of writing this book has been that virtually no scientific trials have been conducted on complementary medicine and cerebral palsy. However, having no scientific evidence is not the same as having no evidence of any kind. The approach of this book is that it is better to use 'unscientific' anecdotal evidence with caution than to say nothing at all.

The information for this book was gathered from as wide a variety of sources as possible. First and foremost it has come from direct contact with disabled people who have experienced complementary medicine. Complementary practitioners and orthodox health professionals have also provided interesting insights and information.

The scientific and medical literature has often proved useful, though often in an indirect manner. For example, research on the mechanisms of acupuncture, though not directly related to cerebral palsy, does give some interesting perspectives of the use of this therapy for the treatment of spasm and other muscle problems. Incidentally, it has been thought inappropriate to include long lists of scientific references in this book. If you are interested in the scientific background to complementary medicine, the book *Complementary Medicine and Disability* (see Further Reading) contains a bibliography with a number of relevant references.

There are various problems in using anecdotes. The most important is that it is difficult to know whether an anecdote is really representative. Practitioners tend to talk about the most interesting and dramatic case histories, even though these will not generally be typical of their everyday case load. Moreover, because cases that are unsuccessful don't usually come back for more treatment, they are easily forgotten. In addition, those people who are most willing to talk about their experiences of complementary medicine are often those who have received the most positive benefits. In sum, the process of conducting the research for this book may have led to subtle biases towards complementary medicine.

This may not be a problem. After all, a standard book

on, say, physiotherapy, aimed at patients and lay people, will generally discuss a series of positive case histories as a means of explaining the scope and end-goal of physiotherapy treatment. This book may be seen in the same light.

The aim of this book is to be *informative* rather than *definitive*. It should be clear from the style of the text that 'what many people have noticed' or 'what is commonly reported' is aiming at giving information to help in the making of practical decisions. This book is not intended to be a final statement of the truth about the role of complementary medicine in cerebral palsy and related conditions.

Acknowledgements

This book is dedicated to Gill Levy, without whose early enthusiasm . . .

Far more people have helped with this project than can be listed here: to all of those who have shared personal experiences, or who have offered help and advice, many thanks. Special mention must go to:

Eileen Milnes, Bob Lister, Raficq Abdulla, Marion Stanton, Kate Nash of the British School of Osteopathy, Eugene Doherty, Maureen Sanderson, Andrew Carman, the CD Family Support Group, Contact a Family.

A proportion of the funding for the background research was provided by Sir Charles Jessel's Charitable Trust and the Research Council for Complementary Medicine.

Duplicated Material

Some material from this book has already been published in *Complementary Medicine and Disability*, Chapman Hall, 1993. The sections that comprise primarily of published material are as follows:

Chapter 1   Self-help or Professional Help.
Chapter 2   Specific and Non-specific Effects of complementary medicine

Chapter 1

Introduction to Complementary Medicine

Complementary therapies involve ideas about health or the body or treatment that are not found in conventional medicine. For example, practitioners of acupuncture believe that health is determined by the state of energy in special pathways in the body; they treat disease by placing needles at special points on the skin. Needless to say, these ideas and methods are not commonly found in orthodox medical practice.

Some people say that over and above not being part of conventional medicine, complementary therapies share a number of common characteristics:

1. *Natural healing.* Complementary practitioners believe that the body has an inherent ability to heal itself and that the aim of treatment should be to stimulate and enhance this capacity. For example, whereas an orthodox practitioner might treat a cold by prescribing an antibiotic to kill off the bacteria causing the infection, a complementary practitioner might focus on strengthening the individual's immune system.
2. *Holistic medicine.* Complementary practitioners say that in looking for the cause and treatment of disease, doctors tend to look only at the physical body. They claim that complementary medicine also involves considering the mental, spiritual and emotional aspects of the individual.

3. *Non-invasive treatment.* Complementary therapies are generally gentle and pleasant: high technology is avoided and negative side-effects are rare.
4. *Client-centred approach.* The relationship between therapist and client is seen to be of prime importance by practitioners of complementary medicine. Moreover, complementary medicine often involves clients becoming active participants in treatment. This involves not only dietary change and the practice of techniques such as meditation or yoga but it also extends to taking personal responsibility for healthcare and to making decisions about how treatment should proceed.

One of the problems of this list of characteristics is that many are also found in orthodox medicine. For example, many doctors are interested in the holistic approach to healthcare and many do encourage their patients to become actively involved in treatment. This has lead at least some people to the conclusion that there is no such thing as complementary medicine. In this view, complementary medicine is just a convenient label to describe a loose collection of disparate therapies.

In the case of disability, however, there is a genuine reason to see complementary medicine as a distinct field. This is so that it might be distinguished from what will be termed 'unorthodox therapies'.

UNORTHODOX THERAPIES

Conductive education, Doman-Delcato and holding therapy are all examples of unorthodox therapies. There are a number of ways of differentiating these unorthodox therapies from complementary medicine.

One of the most general points is that the most unorthodox therapies have been developed specifically for the treatment of certain subgroups of disability. 'Holding therapy', for example, is only used to treat autism; Doman-Delcato is designed to treat children who have brain damage. Complementary therapies have developed as systems of medicine in their own right, so that the use of the therapy with a disabled person represents just one of its possible applications. For example, though osteopathy can be used with young children who have cerebral palsy, it can also be an appropriate treatment for an adult who has arthritis, or insomnia, or who just feels tense and burnt out. It is obviously hard to imagine a fatigued adult turning to conductive education or holding therapy.

An associated point is that whereas most unorthodox therapies are relatively young – the theory behind Doman-Delcato, for example, was born in the 1940s – the majority of complementary therapies have traditions that stretch back many hundreds or thousands of years.

Unorthodox therapies also differ in that they were generally created by orthodox health professionals. Doman-Delcato was developed by a physiotherapist, an educator and a physician; similarly, the originators of Bobath were a physiotherapist and a doctor. Many complementary therapies cannot be attributed to a single creator: the origins of herbal medicine and massage, for example, probably predate human history. In those cases where a complementary therapy was created by an individual, that individual was either not a physician (for example, F.M. Alexander, founder of the Alexander technique) or was not practising what would be currently recognized as medicine (for example, Hahnemann, the founder of homoeopathy, originally used cupping and bleeding to treat patients).

It is also worth pointing out that whereas many of those practising unorthodox therapies have orthodox medical qualifications, often in physiotherapy or occupational therapy, most complementary practitioners are not medically qualified.

However, perhaps the single most important factor that distinguishes complementary from unorthodox medicine is that of medical theory. Complementary therapies often diverge significantly from orthodox medical understanding. For example, acupuncturists believe that health is determined by the flow of energy along special channels that run through the body. Needless to say, this is not a belief that can be found in a standard medical textbook. Fundamental theoretical differences between unorthodox therapies and their orthodox counterparts, on the other hand, are rarely substantial: what restricts their use in conventional settings such as the NHS is primarily the fact that they remain unproven.

Complementary Medicine	*Unorthodox Medicine*
Systems of medicine with wide ranges of application.	Generally specific to a certain category of disability.
Traditional: many complementary therapies were developed thousands of years ago.	Originated in recent history.
Often created, developed and practised by those without orthodox medical qualifications.	Usually created, developed and practised by doctors, physiotherapists and other orthodox health professionals.
Theory may diverge significantly from orthodox scientific beliefs.	Substantial differences with orthodox theory are rare.

This book is concerned with complementary, rather than with unorthodox, therapies. This is not because techniques such as conductive education or Doman-Delcato are somehow 'not as good' as massage, herbal medicine and the rest. It is because there are already sources of advice and information about unorthodox therapies that cater to the needs of people with disabilities and their carers. There is nothing comparable in complementary medicine. For information on unorthodox therapies see Chapter 4.

COMPLEMENTARY MEDICINE DOES NOT REPLACE ORTHODOX MEDICINE

Many of the therapies mentioned in this book are called 'alternative medicine' by some people. This seems to suggest that they are something you might consider instead of seeing your doctor. The term 'complementary' is now favoured by many workers because it suggests that it is, of course, possible to do both: going for a massage, taking up yoga or using homoeopathic remedies are all things which can be done in addition to most treatments suggested by an orthodox physician.

There are a number of different ways in which complementary and conventional medicine can be combined. Firstly, different therapies can be used for entirely different purposes. John, for example, takes regular medication for the respiratory infections to which he is prone. He also visits a massage practitioner and uses a relaxation technique at home, both of which he enjoys and finds relaxing. Similarly, Imran receives physiotherapy and speech therapy at a child development centre. His mother also takes him to an osteopath in the hope that he can be helped to become less irritable and distracted.

Complementary and conventional therapies can also work in tandem on the same health problem. For example, Graham's father takes him to an osteopath to supplement his physiotherapy: his hope is that any improvement in his mobility will be greater with the combination of the two therapies than with either one alone. Likewise, Inez, who takes medication for epilepsy, is taken to an acupuncturist because it is felt that acupuncture treatment might further reduce the frequency of her seizures.

A slight variation is where complementary therapies are used in an attempt to prevent a recurrence of a symptom, though when the symptom does recur, its treatment is left to orthodox medicine. Nell regularly suffers severe flu. She is prescribed a course of homoeopathy with the aim of reducing the frequency of her bouts of flu; however, she will still take antibiotics when she does fall sick.

By combining complementary and orthodox medicine in certain ways, many individuals have managed to get the best of both, utilizing what each has to offer in order to get the maximum benefit.

In Chapter 3, you will find a discussion on how to decide on a programme of healthcare to overcome health problems and maximize general well-being. What appears to be true is that in the majority of cases, the best programmes involve elements of both complementary and orthodox medicine. The two forms of medicine are not competing 'alternatives' – each offers a set of resources that individuals can employ to best effect: complementary medicine does not replace orthodox medicine.

SELF-HELP OR PROFESSIONAL HELP?

Many people seem to think that complementary healthcare is primarily about self-help: in this view, the alternative to the doctor's surgery is the health store, with its bottles of herbal remedies and vitamin pills, and the bookshop, with its *How to . . .* health and diet guides.

The problem is that healthcare is more complicated than a book, or a bottle of pills, might suggest. For example, a health store might sell a herbal tablet for 'arthritis'. However, there are many different types of arthritis and each condition involves symptoms other than joint pain. Moreover, recovery from an arthritic condition may require physiotherapy exercise to improve and maintain mobility.

Similarly, most books on complementary medicine tend

to be rather over simplified. In addition to the many diet guides (each of which claims to be the one true way to perfect health) you will normally find books on homoeopathy and herbal medicine. These generally list remedies for individual complaints: hornbeam for tiredness, peppermint for indigestion, valerian for insomnia and so on. However, prescribing remedies in complementary medicine normally depends on a complex assessment of the individual, rather than on one or two symptoms. Put it this way: if complementary medicine were really as straightforward as self-help books tell us, there would really be no need for registered practitioners to study for three years to learn their trade.

Professional practitioners of medicine have experience and understanding of healthcare. They are also able to offer skilled techniques, such as an osteopathic manipulation to ease a sore back or acupuncture to help with pain. Finally, a practitioner will be able to offer energy and support. Healing can be a long and difficult process and having health problems, or being a carer, can be both physically and emotionally draining. For example, it might be a lot to ask of a parent that they care for a child who had cerebral palsy, lose many nights of sleep, fight the case with social services and be solely responsible for the child's healthcare.

If an individual has a serious problem with his or her health, treatment should involve a professional practitioner. Though self-help has many advantages, and though it often plays an important role in complementary therapy, it should be seen essentially as an additional resource.

Seeking professional help, however, can bring its own problems. Professionals can sometimes act, or be treated by their clients, as 'experts' and they can sometimes take, or be given, power over other people's lives merely on the basis of their technical knowledge. Furthermore, the mere act of consulting a professional may lessen a person's sense of self-reliance and self-worth or a parent's sense of involvement in his or her child's care.

It is important that people who wish to use complementary healthcare are aware of these possibilities. Professionals should be seen as 'enablers', who help individuals to achieve their aims, rather than as experts. This suggests a more equal role for practitioner and client, in fact, some workers describe the ideal relation ship as a 'therapeutic *partnership*' in which mutual trust, empathy and respect are the key elements.

There is some disagreement as to the implications of this in the treatment of children. Some practitioners consider the whole family to be the 'client' so that it is the family that takes responsibility for, and makes decisions about, healthcare and that may become involved in exercise and dietary change. Such practitioners may actively include parents in the decision-making process and in treatment. Some will also give treatments to parents and other members of the family as part of a programme of healthcare for the child.

On the other hand, there are practitioners who prefer to treat children as just another 'case'. They may actually state a preference for the parent to moderate the role they play in treatment on the grounds that it is better to work with a child when there is a one-on-one situation. Such practitioners may also point out that it is easier to concentrate on the therapy, and on the child, if there are as few distractions as possible.

As is so often the case in complementary medicine, there are few right or wrong approaches: it is up to the family to decide which style of therapy they prefer. A further discussion of this subject is given in Chapter 5.

DOES IT WORK?

There are a number of different ways of supporting a claim that a particular therapy is effective. The most common method is to use a case history: 'The patient had symptoms a, b and c, I treated using therapy d and the patient was cured.' The problem with the case history is that there is no way of knowing whether the treatment and cure are related. Would the patient have got better anyway? Did the patient recover as a result of another therapy? Or was it the patient's belief in the treatment rather than the treatment itself that led to the improvement?

This is more than just scepticism for scepticism's sake. If we believed in a therapy solely on the grounds of a successful case history, we would have to believe in every therapy that has ever existed, from black magic and medieval potions, to blood letting, to the discredited surgical techniques of the early part of this century, to modern-day fringe practices such as astrological therapy.

One of the best reasons to believe in a therapy is because it has been supported by a well-conducted scientific trial. Contrary to popular belief, a number of complementary therapies have been subjected to scientific scrutiny with the results published in major medical journals. The weight of evidence suggests that there are good reasons to believe that at least some complementary therapies can be effective in at least some conditions.

Homoeopathy

This is one of the easier therapies to test by what is known as 'double-blind, placebo-controlled trial', the most rigorous method of assessing a therapy, and the standard technique for evaluating orthodox drugs. There have been over one hundred studies on homoeopathy, over 75 per cent of which had a positive result. Even the most carefully conducted studies on homoeopathy have proved favourable. On these grounds, it would seem difficult to assert that homoeopathy is effective only because people have faith in it.

Herbal Medicine

There have been successful, well-conducted trials of a number of different herbal remedies. These include valerian for insomnia, ginger for sea-sickness and fever-few for preventing migraine. One recent trial that has gained considerable attention found that a traditional Chinese herbal remedy is effective for certain types of eczema. Such results should not surprise us: herbal products are the basis for a large number of modern drugs including aspirin, quinine, digitalis and morphine.

Nutritional Medicine

A vast number of studies have investigated the effects of diet on health. Trials of interest here include those that demonstrated that diet can be implicated in eczema, bowel disease, hyperactivity and certain cases of epilepsy. These findings cannot be applied too simplistically to disability. For example, the factors involved in causing hyperactivity in an able-bodied child may be different from those in a child with cerebral palsy, and a diet that would be helpful for one might not be so for the other.

Osteopathy and Chiropractic

There have been a number of trials on osteopathy and chiropractic. Though results have been mixed, the majority are favourable. The largest and most important trial conducted in the UK was published in the *Lancet* and concluded: 'For patients with low back pain ... chiropractic almost certainly confers worthwhile, long-term benefit in comparison with hospital out-patient management. Introducing chiropractic into the NHS should be considered.'

Acupuncture

Though a large number of trials have demonstrated that acupuncture is an effective therapy for pain, considerable debate surrounds acupuncture research. This is because the very nature of acupuncture makes it difficult to design scientific trials. However, one authority has summed up the situation by commenting that the effectiveness of acupuncture 'is greater than would be expected from a placebo', in other words, acupuncture works, and not just because people believe in it. Other trials of acupuncture have demonstrated benefit for asthma, nausea and addiction.

Aromatherapy

A number of the oils used by aromatherapists have been analysed and tested in the laboratory. Many have been shown to produce activity against infection; others have been shown to be of benefit for inflammation and high temperature. In a clinical trial conducted in Australia, a gel containing essential oil of tea-tree was found to be effective in the treatment of acne.

Alexander Technique

Though the Alexander technique has not yet been subject to a rigorous trial, a number of studies have demonstrated benefits such as improved respiratory function, improved pain management and improved posture and balance.

Therapies Involving Relaxation

Many complementary therapies involve touch and relaxation, both of which have been demonstrated by rigorous scientific trials to be beneficial: one authority estimates that there are some 3000 studies demonstrating that relaxation has positive effects on health. Conditions covered by this research include pain, asthma and heart disease. In addition to the anecdotal and circumstantial evidence on touch and health, studies have demonstrated positive effects of massage such as increased weight gain in premature babies and decreased anxiety among adolescents in psychiatric hospitals.

There have been many studies on healing, though the overwhelming majority were not published in major journals. In the USA, healing is used by nurses in orthodox hospitals and has been studied in these settings. One trial found that healing was effective in calming children; another showed an effect on tension headache pain. In Holland, a trial found that healing improved general well-being in people with hypertension. Recently, two well-designed trials appear to demonstrate that healing can be an effective treatment for surgical trauma and wound healing.

There have been few published studies on other complementary therapies.

WHAT CONCLUSIONS CAN BE DRAWN FROM THE DATA ON COMPLEMENTARY MEDICINE?

The first point, and perhaps one of the most important, is that complementary medicine can be indeed scientifically studied. Many people had thought (actually, many still do) that complementary therapies are somehow untestable and 'unscientific', a point of view that prevents any serious discussion of how they might be used in a setting such as the National Health Service. Secondly, given the available evidence, it would seem hard to argue that complementary therapies are effective only because they are 'placebos', in other words, they work only because people believe in them. At least some complementary therapies do appear to have at least some tangible, medical benefits.

That said, it is worth noting that the debate on complementary medicine is far from over. The amount of evidence 'for' complementary medicine is tiny compared to that for more orthodox techniques. Some therapies, such as reflexology, have never been studied. Even for those therapies that have been investigated and shown to be beneficial, such as homoeopathy, the vast majority of the remedies and techniques remain untested.

What does appear to be difficult to doubt, however, is that most people who visit complementary practitioners do appear to be satisfied with the treatment they receive. For example, in a widely quoted survey, *Which?* found that 82 per cent of users of complementary medicine thought that they had improved or been cured; 74 per cent said that they would use complementary medicine again and 69 per cent would recommend it to a friend who had a similar complaint.

Summary: What Is Complementary Medicine?

Complementary medicine is a term that can be used to refer to a number of different therapies, each of which has its own particular principles and practices. As a result, complementary medicine is sometimes described merely as anything that isn't conventional medical practice. However, complementary therapies do happen to share a number of common characteristics:

- The belief that therapies should work with the inherent healing capacities of the body.
- A gentle and generally pleasant form of treatment.
- A natural and open relationship between practitioner and client.

- An active role for the client.
- A complementary rather than an alternative relationship to conventional medicine.
- Theories and practices that diverge from current scientific understanding.

There are also some things that complementary medicine is not:

- Complementary therapy is not a replacement for orthodox medicine: it should be used in addition, rather than as an alternative, to the therapies recommended by orthodox practitioners.
- Complementary medicine does not include the specialist therapies, such as conductive education and Doman-Delcato.
- Complementary medicine should not be confused with the self-help available at your local health store: the complementary treatment of serious conditions, such as cerebral palsy, should generally involve a professional practitioner.
- Complementary medicine is not untested. There have been several rigorous scientific trials that suggest that certain complementary therapies can be of benefit in at least some conditions.

Chapter 2

What Can Complementary Medicine Do?

Many people don't know what to expect from complementary medicine. Some seem to hope for some sort of cure, and a quick one at that. With this view, the effects of complementary medicine are all-or-nothing: either the client resumes a totally normal life after a course of treatment or he or she receives no benefit at all. The idea that complementary medicine is all about 'miracle cures' has been encouraged by the media:

> After his first . . . treatment, a 15-year-old boy was able to read whole words for the first time.

Given that many thousands of practitioners give many millions of consultations every year, it is perhaps not surprising that, every so often, a case comes up that is suitably 'newsworthy'. However, dramatic cures do not reflect the general experience of people who use complementary therapies and there are a number of reasons why it may be advisable to forget about miracle cures. Not only does disappointment have a generally negative and depressing effect but many practitioners have come to the conclusion that complementary therapies become most effective when the client and family play an active and involved role in a programme of treatment: looking for miracles means lying back and letting some outside agent do the work.

There are a number of other things worth saying about the effects of complementary medicine.

1. *Complementary medicine is not a cure for cerebral palsy.* Cerebral palsy cannot be cured by complementary or any other form of medicine simply because cerebral palsy involves damage to the nervous system. This cannot be reversed. Complementary therapies do sometimes lead to significant improvements in some children. However, these improvements are not total.

2. *The results of complementary treatment depend on the therapy concerned.* It may seem obvious to point out that massage and homoeopathy aim to do very different things, but it is surprising how many people forget this when they ask whether 'complementary medicine' could help a certain problem. In Chapter 4 there is a description of the effects of a number of different therapies. These range from gentle relaxation (for example, as found in massage) to the control of secondary symptoms such as constipation (homoeopathy) to changes in mobility and function (acupuncture).

3. *Complementary medicine takes time before its effects are felt.* Most practitioners believe that their techniques work by stimulating the body's own natural self-repair systems and this process, of course, takes time. Imagine an arrowhead in a wound: it is clear that removing the arrowhead will allow the wound to heal, but this still might take a number of months to happen. So whereas the time needed for say, a drug, to have an effect is generally measured in hours and days, complementary therapies tend to require weeks and months before any benefit is seen.

4. *The effects of complementary medicine are not restricted to particular symptoms or health problems.* The technical way of putting this is to say that complementary therapies can have both *specific* and *non-specific* effects.

SPECIFIC AND NON-SPECIFIC EFFECTS OF COMPLEMENTARY THERAPIES

Althea has recurrent colds and flu. Her mother takes her to a homoeopath who prescribes a homoeopathic remedy and suggests a change to her diet. As a result, Althea's respiratory infections gradually diminish towards a more normal level. Barry tries a course of reflexology treatments on the advice of a friend. He feels calm and relaxed after each session and says that he has much more energy than he used to.

Althea experienced what is known as a *specific* effect of therapy, when a particular symptom or health problem improves. Barry, on the other hand, experienced *non-specific* or *generalized* effects: though he 'feels better' in himself, he finds it difficult to point to individual symptoms that no longer worry him.

Conventional medicine traditionally concentrates on specific effects. For example, a doctor might treat athlete's foot with an anti-fungal skin cream. The aim in this case is very specific: to eradicate the fungus and thereby relieve the symptoms of pain and itching.

Complementary therapies are found at the opposite end of the spectrum. Almost everyone who tries a therapy says that they feel 'better in themselves' or that they have a 'general sense of well-being'. Often, however, they may find it difficult to identify the exact way in which they feel better and specific health problems may be left unchanged.

Within complementary medicine, different therapies vary as to the degree to which their effects are specific or generalized. Massage, healing, meditation and yoga are good examples of techniques where the outcome of treatment is generalized; acupuncture, osteopathy and homoeopathy are examples of therapies that have more specific effects. There is much crossover however: people who have successful osteopathic treatment often experience an improved sense of well-being; conversely massage, and even yoga and meditation, can be used for specific symptoms.

It is important to think about the difference between specific and non-specific effects of treatment. When many people ask the question: 'What will complementary medicine do for me (or my child)?' they often expect the answer to be in terms of improved physical function, recovery from illness or increased mental ability (specific effects of treatment). It is often seen as somehow weak and irrelevant if an answer is in terms of more generalized effects, for example, feelings of well-being and self-esteem or being able to better cope with pain.

The prejudice can be extremely damaging, especially when disability is involved. In some cases, significant improvements in walking, speech, hand function and so on may not be possible. However, this does not mean that the individual's quality of life cannot be enhanced. It is not uncommon for parents to be so set on trying to 'fix' their child's disability that some potential benefits of therapy, such as general feelings of well-being or increased motivation, are entirely forgotten.

Non-Specific Effects of Complementary Medicine

General Well-being

Many people have found that complementary therapy has led to improved general well-being. One of the most common phrases used is 'I feel so much better in myself'. Some people feel a sense of inner calm and peace of mind; others feel something like euphoria ('I feel bubbly'); many experience both.

Many of those who try complementary treatment also say that they feel more positive, motivated and assured:

> Since the treatment, I have been much more confident, more stable, and better able to take charge of life.

The comments that many parents make about their children after complementary therapy mirror these remarks.

The single most common observation is: 'He always used to be sickly and unwell. He's so much healthier and stronger and cheerful now.'

Another important consideration is that most complementary therapies are pleasurable and deeply relaxing. Many of the comments that disabled people have made about complementary therapies make reference to how good it helped them feel: 'Though I am paralysed from the waist down, Alexander lessons make me fly'; 'After massage I feel on top of the world'; 'It makes me feel wonderful.' For someone who has found their body a source of frustration, and perhaps of pain, the realization that it can also be a source of pleasure and relaxation can be profoundly important.

Some parents have described complementary treatment sessions as a 'special time emotionally' for their children. Often, the child relaxes totally and falls asleep during treatment. It is also common for the child to lie very still and concentrate on the treatment, sometimes with a small smile. Older children may relate that therapy 'feels good'. Several parents have pointed out that this can be particularly important because therapy normally 'feels bad': the techniques that physiotherapists use are generally unpleasant, and often painful, and hospitals and surgery are widely recognized to be harrowing experiences for a child.

Self-image

A significant number of disabled people have problems with the image they have of their own body: they may see themselves as ugly or deformed, and there may be the feeling that: 'My body has let me down.' There may be anger at the body, a frustration at opportunities missed because things weren't different. As a counsellor for disabled people summed it up: 'A large proportion of the clients I see positively hate their own body.'

There can be little doubt that many of these feelings

have been engendered by a society that handicaps people whose bodies fall outside a certain norm by the emplacement of social, physical and legislative barriers and that produces a popular fiction that often associates moral weakness with physical stigmata.

Improved self-image is a common consequence of complementary healthcare. One of the most commonly cited reasons for this is that many of the therapies involve touch. This touch is quite distinct from the nurse's or care worker's lifting manoeuvres, or from the physiotherapist's stretching and manipulating; it is a more gentle, human touch, one that communicates calmness and acceptance. As one massage practitioner put it:

> Sometimes I just hold the client's head or arm gently in my hands. It's a way of saying "This is how you are". You can feel when someone relaxes into it.

Some people have noticed that increased self-acceptance is a common consequence of complementary medicine, especially among disabled people. An associated point is that complementary medicine can sometimes lead to an appreciation of our non-physical aspects:

> Meditation put me in touch with myself. And I discovered that I was not my physical body, that I was not equal to, and bound by, this thing that other people called "deformed".

Tension, Relaxation and Calmness

Many complementary therapies are particularly good at bringing about a profound sense of relaxation, something that is not only pleasant, but very health-promoting. Feelings of calmness and relaxation are not restricted to the actual treatment session, they may last for several days or weeks; some people find that they are even more long-lasting: 'I'm not a tense person any more, before I was really tense.' The physical side effects of relaxation can include improved sleep patterns and decreased pain and spasm.

The ability of complementary therapies to relax and calm irritable and distracted children is seen by many parents as its number one benefit. Complementary therapy generally takes place in calming and soothing environments, and many people find that the practitioner has a quieting effect on their child:

It was very peaceful in his room. Tracy stopped crying as soon as he picked her up.

He's so calming. I relax a lot, and perhaps that's the reason my son starts to relax.

Treatment itself is often very soothing. The therapies that involve touch have particularly calming effects:

She falls asleep as soon as she touches the treatment table.

I'm amazed that he lies there so still for so long. He won't normally remain in one spot for more than about a minute.

She was screaming and crying when we went to see the practitioner. When we brought her back to the car, she was fast asleep.

Most parents find that any soothing and calming effects last at least a few hours or days after treatment. A common experience is that the child tends to sleep well, the night following a treatment. Some parents also find that the changes are more long lasting.

He's definitely less irritable nowadays.

At night she'd cry and wouldn't sleep, and in the day she'd be all irritable and angry. The problem cleared completely after the treatment.

Specific Effects of Complementary Medicine

In addition to non-specific or generalized effects on well-being, such as those outlined above, complementary therapies can be effective at remedying specific symptoms. In this respect, it is important to make a distinction between *primary* and *secondary* symptoms. Primary symptoms are the main health problems caused by a particular condition. In cerebral palsy, the primary symptom is motor deficit, simply speaking, difficulties with movement. Other primary symptoms can include spasticity or involuntary movements (depending on the type of cerebral palsy) and sometimes hearing or visual impairment.

Secondary symptoms are described as such because they result not so much from the underlying condition, but from some associated process. Any particular individual may have all, some or none of the secondary symptoms; moreover, many secondary symptoms are relatively common in people who do not have the condition in question.

A pressure sore is a good example of a secondary symptom. Pressure sores are not a direct result of any particular illness or disability, but are caused by sitting in a wheelchair or lying in bed over a period of time. Constipation is another example of a secondary symptom: constipation in children with cerebral palsy is caused by a combination of factors that include lowered intake of food (due to a lower requirement) and lowered mobility of the gut (caused by problems of abdominal muscle tone and low general mobility.)

It is worth pointing out that there is no hard and fast distinction between primary and secondary symptoms. In fact, what is a primary symptom for one person may be a secondary for another: for example, learning disability is a primary symptom in at least some children with cerebral palsy; however, there are others for whom learning disability results not so much from direct damage to the brain, but from physical and sensory impairments, and from poor teaching and lack of stimulation. A further complication is that something that improves a secondary symptom may well have a knock on effect on a primary symptom. For example, children who suffer recurrent colds are not generally at their best as far as learning motor and intellectual skills are concerned and, as a result, any remedy that reduces the frequency of the colds will be of more general benefit to the child's development.

Examples of the Effects of Complementary Healthcare

Specific Effects	*Non-specific Effects*
Stronger walking	General feelings of well-being
Increased joint mobility	'The pain is still there, but it doesn't bother me so much'
Improved speech	Relaxation, calmness and improved sleep
Recovery from infection	Increased motivation; feeling positive about life
Improved bowel and bladder function	'I feel in touch with myself'

In this book, problems with physical mobility and learning will be considered to be primary symptoms. Listed below are some of the problems that are secondary problems, and that are most commonly reported to be helped by complementary treatment. Obviously, being disabled does not mean having any health problems at all, so you will have to decide which, if any, of these apply to you or your child. This is just a brief overview: more information on the effects of complementary therapy can be found in Chapter 4.

Recurrent Infections

Complementary medicine can sometimes be effective for recurrent infections. Practitioners say that this is because complementary therapy can strengthen the immune system. In a typical case parents might notice that their child had far fewer colds in the winter following a course of say, osteopathy, than during the previous winter. In addition to infections of the respiratory tract, complementary practitioners have also treated gastric and urinary infections and 'glue ear' (otitis media).

Digestion and Appetite

Users of complementary medicine often report improved appetite and a decreased incidence of problems such as indigestion or heartburn. Some practitioners have commented that such benefits are especially common in cerebral palsy. This may be due to an improvement in the muscle tone of the abdomen.

Bowels and Bladder

An improvement in bowel or bladder function is one of the most commonly reported effects of complementary medicine. Constipation appears to be particularly susceptible to complementary treatment, as does infantile colic.

Pain

Some people who have experienced pain relief through complementary medicine say that though the pain is still there, it doesn't bother them so much: the physical sensation is less unpleasant and the pain places fewer restrictions on their activities and enjoyment of life. Others have noticed a significant decrease in the amount of pain they experience and this is often because the cause of the pain, for example constipation, has been treated successfully.

Spasm, Spasticity and Other Involuntary Movements

Many complementary therapies can bring about relaxation. This is thought to be of benefit for muscle tone and for involuntary movements such as athetosis. There is also evidence that some therapies, particularly acupuncture, can have a specific effect on spasm.

Behavioural Problems

As pointed out in the preface, this book will only cover problems such as hyperactivity where they are associated with a physical disability such as cerebral palsy. Many complementary therapies are very relaxing, and relaxation does appear to be effective at moderating a variety of behavioural problems. Though this is generally a short-term effect, it is not unknown for more profound and long-term changes to occur.

Communication Difficulties

Many complementary therapies involve touch and, as such, they can be used as a means of communication, particularly for certain groups of people with learning disabilities.

Skin Problems

A number of complementary therapies can be useful in conditions such as eczema or dry skin.

Epilepsy

Complementary medicine has proved effective at reducing frequency and severity of seizures in some cases. However, epilepsy is a complex condition and individual variation to treatment is high.

THE EFFECTS OF COMPLEMENTARY MEDICINE ON MOBILITY AND LEARNING DISABILITY

When discussing the effects of any form of therapy on mobility and learning disability, it is worth making the distinction between short-term and long-term change. Often, treatments bring about change for only a few hours or days after a session. For example, John, who has cerebral palsy, finds that a good message loosens him up so that walking, sitting and talking are easier. However, he finds that these benefits wear off during the week, at the end of which he says he is: 'Back to normal'.

John's experience is extremely common. Many therapies are able to bring about short-term improvements across a wide range of conditions, something that is attributable, at least in part, to the 'placebo effect'. This is one of the reasons why many people feel that the only real test of a therapy is its long-term outcome. For example, most parents would like to know whether putting their children through a course of therapy will make any difference to their ability to walk or talk in later life. Unfortunately, answering that question involves considerable difficulties.

Effects on Mobility and Learning Disability: Children

It is very important to point out that no one really knows whether complementary medicine can bring about long-term improvements in physical and learning disability in children. The simple reason for this is that no rigorous medical trials have been conducted, and though rigorous medical trials are not the only way of finding out about healthcare, they are certainly one of the best ways we have of generating information that is reliable.

Evidence for the effects of complementary therapies on disabled children comes largely from anecdotal reports. The problem with anecdotes is that it is always possible to wonder whether it was really the therapy that caused the changes or whether they would have happened anyway. Another problem is that most children are undergoing a number of different therapies at the same time. It is often difficult to know which therapy caused which effect.

To give a practical example: a child with cerebral palsy visits a cranial osteopath. After a few treatments, the parents notice that the child is sitting more strongly and that he seems more bright and alert. However, the child is also having physiotherapy and visiting a conductive education centre. How can we know whether it was the osteopathy that brought about the improvements and not some perhaps delayed effect of another therapy? And what about the possibility that none of the therapies had any effect at all, and that the child would have developed the new abilities without medical intervention?

Even given these difficulties and complications, however, a number of points do seem to be clear.

1. *Short-term improvements can lead to long-term benefit.* This is the rationale of much physiotherapy. For example, a physiotherapist may work to loosen the muscles in a child's limb. Though the effect may only be temporary, such treatment does make it easier for the child to use the limb and this in turn improves its strength and suppleness.

   As has already been noted, complementary therapies appear to be particularly effective in controlling secondary symptoms such as recurrent infection or constipation. It is clear that a child who has painful constipation, or who is down with flu, will not be at his or her best for the learning of intellectual or motor skills. To use an analogy: few people would consider studying a book, or learning to juggle, on days when they were sick. Complementary therapies might lead to long-term benefit by controlling short-term symptoms.

2. *Certain complementary therapies appear to bring about long-term improvements in physical functioning in at least some children.* There is increasing anecdotal evidence that osteopathy and acupuncture can lead to physical improvements that are maintained in the long term. There are a number of reasons why, despite its drawbacks, this evidence seems to warrant a positive, if cautious, conclusion.

Firstly, the number of cases in which disabled children have apparently shown sustained benefit after osteopathy or acupuncture treatment is relatively large. In short, success stories are not just a one-off.

Secondly, the nature of the improvements seems to indicate that they were a direct result of the complementary therapy. For example, if a child has been undergoing a variety of orthodox therapies for a continuous period and then experiences an improvement shortly after the commencement of osteopathy, it is tempting to ascribe the improvement to the introduction of this new therapy. Another typical case is where the parents and teacher of a child notice a sudden and unprecedented improvement a couple of days after a particular treatment session.

Thirdly, practitioners interested in research have been documenting case histories with increasing care and sophistication. Some have even gone as far as comparing the progress of a group receiving complementary therapy with a control group that received no treatment. Though such research is open to criticism, the documented results are certainly difficult to explain away.

3. *The long-term effects of complementary therapy on learning disability and on social and emotional problems are unclear.* It

is widely acknowledged that problems such as learning disability or behavioural disorder are not only more difficult to assess than physical disability but also more prone to be affected by factors outside a practitioner's control. For example, a change of school or social worker, or a resolution of family difficulties can have dramatic effects on an individual's intellectual and emotional well-being. Moreover, intellectual and emotional development is less predictable than physical development: take the fact that there is greater variation in the age at which children start to speak than there is in the age at which they start to walk. Finally, intellectual and emotional development is dependent, at least partly, on physical functioning: physical disabilities such as impaired hand function, or recurring illnesses such as flu, can complicate the learning of intellectual and social skills.

It is not surprising then that the effects of complementary therapy on learning disability and emotional problems are open to debate, even among practitioners. For example, as pointed out on pages 92–3, whereas some acupuncture practitioners say that they are able to improve mental ability in some disabled children, other practitioners are sceptical of these claims. That said, some of the well-documented case histories (see above) do indicate improvements in learning disability and in emotional and social problems. Improvements in behaviour appear to be most common in osteopathic treatment.

4. *Complementary therapies do not provide a cure.* If we accept that complementary therapies can sometimes lead to significant improvements in at least some children, it must be pointed out that these improvements are not total. Typical examples of improvements attributed to complementary medicine might be: the ability to stand with support having previously been unable to stand; the ability to use single words; the ability to load a spoon before feeding. Often, though one area of func-

tion is improved, another remains unaffected. For example, a child may stop drooling and experience fewer seizures yet might remain unable to walk independently. Even in the more remarkable cases given by complementary practitioners, the children involved remain disabled to some degree.

5. *The extent of improvement is related to the severity of the symptoms and the age of the child.* In general, the milder a set of symptoms, the easier they are to control. Just as a mild headache will respond more readily to aspirin than a severe migraine, so the severity of a child's disabilities will affect the degree to which a complementary practitioner is able to bring about positive improvements.

Another medical generalization is that young children respond more readily to treatment than older children. Complementary practitioners say that the earlier the treatment is started, the better. For example, one acupuncturist has reported that his work is very much more effective in those who are 5 years or younger than in those who are older than 6 years. That said, at least some practitioners have reported improvements in adolescents and adults.

Effects on Mobility and Learning Disability: Adolescents and Adults

The effects of complementary medicine in adults are less dramatic, and of shorter duration, than in children. Cases in which adults have gained new abilities after a course of complementary therapy are extremely rare. Typically, an individual might find something they are already able to do somewhat easier ('My speech is a little clearer and I am walking more steadily'). However, such benefits are often short term and may depend on continuing treatment. For most adults, complementary therapy has been beneficial in terms of quality of life, rather than in terms of improved function. In Chapter 4, you will find examples of the way in which some adults and older children have benefited from complementary medicine.

DISADVANTAGES OF COMPLEMENTARY MEDICINE

This chapter has attempted to answer the question: 'What can complementary medicine do?' This has inevitably led to a list of potential benefits of complementary medicine. However, complementary medicine also has a number of negative features and disadvantages, particularly when compared with orthodox medicine.

1. Whereas conventional therapy is generally available free of charge on the NHS, complementary medicine must usually be paid for directly by the client.
2. There is less control over the competence of practitioners in complementary medicine: the well-known problem of quackery.
3. Complementary medicine is not generally as readily available as orthodox medicine. Unlike a bottle of sleeping pills or headache tablets, complementary therapy cannot usually be kept to hand to be used as and when required.
4. Most conventional therapies can be relied upon to have at least some positive benefit: sleeping pills do usually help a person to fall asleep and headache tablets do normally reduce head pain. The response of an individual to complementary medicine is far less predictable.
5. There are some things that are beyond the scope of complementary medicine. For example, no complementary therapy is able to replace blood lost from a wound or replace a damaged joint.

Complementary Healthcare Is Not Always Successful

Sometimes, a course of complementary treatment does not result in any significant benefit. Though complementary therapy may fail altogether – for example, a person might try homoeopathy for cystitis and experience no improvement at all – it is perhaps more common for an individual to gain some sort of benefit, though not enough to make the time and expense of healthcare worthwhile. For example, someone might find that reflexology makes them feel very relaxed and well in themselves for a few hours after each session, but after a number of treatments they may realize that they have experienced only marginal relief from some of their most troublesome symptoms.

It is not unusual for a person to try a number of different practitioners and therapies before finding a combination that works for them (see also page 45). You should not expect complementary healthcare always to be successful: your own experiences may well be mixed, with perhaps some of the things you try not being fully worth the time, money and effort you may have invested in them.

'There's Nothing Wrong With Not Doing Complementary Medicine'

Some people feel pressured to try complementary therapies. It is not uncommon for friends to repeatedly mention therapies they've heard about ('A colleague of Mrs D. has taken her daughter and it's had the most amazing effects.') and the implicit and often unwanted suggestion is that 'you too should try it'. Simply reading about complementary medicine – this book, for example – can often have a similar effect.

Another prevalent assumption is that if you or your child has a health problem or disability you should try absolutely everything possible to 'get better'. In some social groups there can also be a strange form of inverted snobbery about healthcare: people who try alternative medicine are seen as adventurous and empowered, whereas those who stick to conventional medicine are seen as unimaginative and somewhat incapable.

The comment that forms the title of this section was made by the coordinator of a parent's support group. She says that she has met many parents who have spent years taking their child off to dozens of different therapists. These parents often forget, understandably, that there is more to life than therapy, and that time and effort can also be profitably spent on just playing with and getting to know a child. Moreover, spending a high proportion of time in medical environments can reinforce a child's perception of themselves as being different: as sick and disabled.

In a similar vein, a well-known paediatrician has identified a number of psychological reasons why parents of disabled children have a propensity to visit practitioners of unconventional therapies. For example, some parents feel angry at orthodox medicine: partly because it has failed to provide a cure and partly because it is a natural impulse to shoot the messenger who brings the bad news. This doctor feels that complementary medicine may well have a role in the care of children with conditions such as cerebral palsy. He does believe, however, that it is important for parents to identify rationally the reasons for their interest in complementary medicine.

In short, there shouldn't be any 'shoulds' about complementary medicine. You might well read this book and feel that complementary therapy is not something you would be interested in pursuing. If so, be aware that you may sometimes feel under pressure to change your mind.

Summary: What Can Complementary Medicine Do?

- Complementary medicine is not a cure for cerebral palsy.
- Each complementary therapy has different aims and methods: what you should expect from complementary medicine depends on the therapy you are trying.

- Complementary medicine often leads to non-specific benefits such as relaxation, general feelings of well-being and improved mood.
- Specific benefits, that is, improvements in particular symptoms, may also be brought about by complementary techniques. Many individuals and parents have especially noticed improvements in 'secondary' problems, for example, recurrent colds or constipation.
- Much controversy surrounds the issue of whether complementary therapies can lead to long-term improvements in 'primary' symptoms, such as walking or learning.
- It does seem that at least some children experience persisting improvements in physical and mental functioning, particularly after acupuncture and osteopathy.
- Long-term improvements in primary symptoms are unusual in adults and older children.
- Complementary medicine is not always successful and it does have a number of disadvantages, especially when compared with orthodox medicine.
- Individuals should not feel that they are obliged to try complementary medicine, even though they may come under pressure to do so.

Chapter 3

How to Choose a Therapy and Practitioner

People who are considering complementary medicine often worry about quackery: they wonder how they can be sure that a practitioner is competent or that a therapy is safe and effective. But deciding on complementary medicine is actually a two-stage process: firstly, you do have to ask:

- Are the therapy and practitioner safe and reputable and do I have a reasonable chance of success?

Then you have to ask:

- Is this combination of therapy and practitioner the right one for me or my child?

Making decisions about complementary medicine is not merely a case of avoiding quacks, it is also about positive choices of what you really want from healthcare and a means by which you can maximize your chance of success.

In this respect, complementary medicine is little different from other decisions you have to make. Take choosing a cottage holiday from a brochure: firstly, you have to make sure that the tour operator is reputable and that they won't take your money and 'fly-by-night'. You also have to make sure that the cottages are somewhere pleasant to visit: in a seaside village, for example, rather than an industrial estate. But once you are sure that your holiday is basically safe and sound, you will still want to consider which particular cottage you would like to rent for your holiday.

How Do I Avoid Quacks?

Choose Your Therapy with Care

One of the main ways of avoiding quacks is to stick to safe and reputable therapies. If you steer well clear of fringe and unusual techniques you will be cutting out a large proportion of those who practise without requisite skills and knowledge. Many authorities on the subject say that the majority of quacks use techniques such as crystals, aura diagnosis and astrology, rather than homoeopathy, acupuncture and osteopathy.

The question of which therapies are safe and reputable is answered in Chapter 4. A number of different criteria have been used in choosing the therapies described in this book.

1. *The therapy must be known to be safe and appropriate* – in some cases at least, for people with cerebral palsy and related conditions.
2. *Progress* must be discernible when reviewing the history of the therapy. For example, since it was founded in the late nineteenth century, chiropractic has gained increasing acceptance from the legal and medical authorities; scientific evidence indicating its value has also accumulated and there are ever increasing numbers of practitioners using the technique.
3. *Interest from the medical profession* was also a factor in choosing the therapies. A large number of doctors, nurses, physiotherapists and so on are developing an interest in, and even practising, complementary therapies. Few are using therapies other than those mentioned in the main text of this book. For example, whereas there are NHS homoeopathic hospitals, and

whereas acupuncture is widely available in orthodox pain clinics, crystals and reincarnation therapy have not, as yet, found a foothold in the NHS.

4. *Positive scientific evidence* was seen as an important criterion in choosing therapies (see page 8). Most of the therapies in this book have some form of scientific validation, whereas some of those not mentioned have failed under scientific investigation.

Not every therapy chosen fulfils every criteria. Reflexology, for example, has not been subject to scientific scrutiny; similarly, the history of Rolfing (see page 109) is perhaps too short for it to be worth evaluating the therapy's progress over the course of time. That said, the list of therapies to be included in this book has been evaluated and approved by experts at Scope. As such, using therapies listed in Chapter 4 might well be seen as a useful first step in avoiding quackery.

Make Use of the Professional Registers

Even in the more accepted complementary therapies, there are some practitioners who work without appropriate training and qualifications. One of the best ways to find a competent practitioner is to make use of a professional register. In some therapies, a governing body has managed to establish broad agreement on what skills and knowledge are needed to practise the therapy competently. Individuals meeting standards set out by the governing body are placed on a register and members of the public can then use this register to find capable practitioners. Some organizations have computerized registers and can give you names and addresses over the phone; others can send you a printed copy of their register by post. Details of the contact addresses for the registers are given after each therapy in Chapter 4.

One organization that holds a register for a number of different therapies is the Institute for Complementary

Medicine (see also page 178). The British Register of Complementary Practitioners, as it is known, has not, however, gained widespread approval within complementary medicine. In addition, at the current time of writing, the number of practitioners on the register is relatively small, so though this is sometimes a useful resource, it is certainly not a 'cure all'.

Check Your Practitioner for Yourself

Some therapies do not have a single governing body. A common result of this is that there are often a number of different registers, each with its own set of entry requirements. If there is no broad agreement on standards, there is clearly no easy way to tell who is a competent practitioner and who is not: whereas there may be some qualifications that are worth watching for, others may be barely worth the paper they are written on. Regardless, many excellent practitioners advertise no qualifications at all.

There are a number of therapies for which finding a practitioner may not be a simple case of checking a register:

- massage and aromatherapy
- healing
- reflexology
- nutrition
- disciplines such as meditation, yoga and tai chi

Registers do exist for each of these (see the relevant sections in Chapter 4) but they either fail to include some competent practitioners or fail to set high enough standards. These registers might best be seen as a useful source of appropriate contacts rather than as a means of guaranteeing therapeutic competence.

There may be times when you are not sure of your practitioner's competence, particularly if he or she is using a therapy for which there is not a single register. In such cases, you will have to check the practitioner for yourself.

This is less difficult than it sounds: you just have to look for a few danger signals and ask a few simple questions.

Checking Your Practitioner: Things to Watch Out For

A good rule of thumb in complementary medicine is: 'The more a practitioner promises, the less they will be able to provide.' So, for example, it is a bad sign if your practitioner guarantees you a cure, or promises that your whole life will be put right, or pronounces his or her brilliance from the rooftops. Also watch out for unsolicited offers of therapy, where you are approached in person or by phone.

It can be a good idea to ask a few simple questions. These might include:

- the institute at which the practitioner was trained
- the length of the course
- whether it was full or part-time
- whether or not the practitioner has professional indemnity insurance

Finally, you can ask the practitioner what other therapies might be worthwhile, and to whom he or she would refer you if treatment did not prove to be successful. A practitioner's answer to this question can often be a useful gauge of their personality. It is a good sign if the practitioner answers openly and calmly and has a number of suggestions of where else to find help. It is a bad sign if the answer is confusing and evasive, particularly if emphasis is placed upon the practitioner's success rate and brilliance and how unnecessary it is to look anywhere else.

Many people have problems with this advice in that they feel it would be embarrassing to appear to distrust a practitioner. There are two things worth saying about this. Firstly, you will normally have your first contact with a practitioner on the telephone (see page 44). Distance normally makes things a little easier, moreover, you would not be in the situation of having to turn down a practitioner straight to his or her face (just say 'I'm ringing a few people, I'll call back'). Secondly, most good practitioners are aware of the problems of quackery and are more than happy to spend time reassuring a potential client.

Finally, there is no need to be suspicious of everyone. Making a wrong decision is unlikely to lead to disaster, especially if you follow the advice in Chapter 5 about what should not happen during treatment.

FINDING A COMPETENT PRACTITIONER

Perhaps the best way of looking for a practitioner with appropriate skills and training is to use a professional register. Some registers have stringent entry requirements and guarantee a practitioner's competence; others should be seen more as a useful first step. If you are not using a register, there are other ways of finding a practitioner – some recommended and some not. Recommended ways include:

1. *Advice from friends and colleagues:* many people see this as the ideal way of meeting a health professional.
2. *Asking your GP.* Though GPs are often seen as negative towards complementary medicine, many are happy to give referrals to appropriate local practitioners.
3. *Contacting a local natural health centre.* Natural health centres typically offer a number of different therapies, with each practitioner hiring a room privately. Unless associated with health and beauty, most of these centres are a good first bet.
4. *Ask for information at a local health store.* Many practitioners put their cards up at health food shops.
5. *Contacting a registered practitioner of a different therapy.* You could, for example, find the name of your local osteopath from the register of osteopaths and ask if they know of a good local aromatherapist.
6. *Yellow Pages.* This can sometimes be a help, however,

anyone, regardless of training can get themselves listed.

Ways to find a practitioner that are not recommended include:

1. Visiting natural healing fairs and festivals.
2. Looking for adverts in magazines and newspapers (reputable yoga and meditation courses are, however, advertised in the press).
3. Responding to anything that resembles 'hawking', such as leaflets under the door, mail shots, bill posters or direct approaches in person or by phone.

Most reputable practitioners clearly do not need to resort to any of these approaches. Just as it is commonly said that people who talk the most at parties are the ones who are often the most nervous and uncomfortable, practitioners with the loudest voices are often those with the least skills.

Avoiding Quacks: a Three-Stage Process

1. Choose your therapy with care.
2. Make use of the professional registers.
3. Check the practitioner for yourself.

HOW TO FIND THE RIGHT THERAPY AND
PRACTITIONER: THE IMPORTANCE OF PERSONAL
PREFERENCE

The overall theme of this chapter has been that decisions on complementary medicine involve a two-stage process. Having dealt with the question of how to find a safe and reputable therapy and practitioner, it is now worth discussing how to find the therapy and practitioner that suits the individual.

In conventional medicine, the main task of the doctor is to match up a specific disease with a specific treatment. It is partly as a result of this that we tend to think of health-care in terms of 'one pill: one ill' and in complementary medicine, people have a tendency therefore to ask: 'Which therapy is best for my particular complaint?'

Complementary therapies should not generally be chosen on the basis of symptoms. In fact, what is normally most important is for the individual client or parent to choose a therapy that he or she thinks will be helpful. There are a number of reasons for this. Many complementary therapies are appropriate across a wide range of conditions: a good massage, for example, can be of benefit to almost anyone; acupuncture, as a complete system of medicine, is used to diagnose and treat a vast range of conditions.

Also, the effectiveness of treatment depends at least partly on the individual's belief that it will work. This is what doctors call the 'Placebo effect'. One consequence of the placebo effect is that healthcare tends to be more effective if it is chosen by the client, who will obviously choose the therapy believed to be most beneficial and the practitioner believed to be most likely to help. In conventional medicine, however, this is rarely possible: only someone with medical training can be expected to understand which therapy is most appropriate for a particular diagnosis; moreover, people do not normally have much say in the doctor they are sent to. In complementary medicine, there are no set therapies for specific problems and there is normally a large choice of practitioners available. As a result, personal preference can come to play a more important role.

The final point is that different complementary therapies aim to do very different things, in very different ways. Compare yoga and nutritional therapy: yoga is a self-help technique which, though it can be helpful for a variety of conditions, is not usually used as a specific cure; nutritional therapy, on the other hand, is typically used only as means to correct specific symptoms. An individual's choice of a complementary therapy depends primarily on what they are looking for from healthcare. If, for example, a person is looking for something they can do for themselves, they would be better off choosing meditation or tai chi than osteopathy. If on the other hand they were looking for something that was primarily a deeply relaxing experience, they might think first of massage, healing or shiatsu. However, if the relief of a specific troublesome symptom was a priority, acupuncture or homoeopathy may be the most appropriate therapy.

In making decisions about complementary medicine, your priority should be to:

1. Choose a therapy that you feel is appropriate to your needs.
2. Choose a therapy that you believe would be helpful.
3. Find a practitioner with whom you feel you could develop a positive relationship.

The importance of this last point cannot be over-emphasized: many authorities say that a person's relationship with his or her practitioner is the single most significant factor affecting the outcome of a course of treatment.

Choosing a Suitable Practitioner

Finding the right practitioner, like finding a marital partner, is something that will always depend ultimately on personal choice. But there are some pointers to what you should look for. When considering any practitioner, you might ask yourself a number of questions:

1. Do you trust the practitioner and have faith in their integrity, honesty and ability?
2. Do you feel that you could confide in the practitioner?
3. Do you feel that you could form an equal relationship with this practitioner or do you sense that he or she would wield power over you?

4. Would the practitioner be prepared to admit 'I don't know' or acknowledge weaknesses in knowledge or skills?
5. Will the practitioner suggest self-care or refer you to other practitioners if the need arose?
6. Will the practitioner help you set your own goals and agenda or try to impose his or her own upon you?
7. Do you feel the practitioner will treat you with respect and dignity?
8. Does the practitioner make you feel hopeful and strengthen your expectations that you or your child can be helped?
9. Would you prefer the practitioner to be of a certain gender or age? Is the practitioner's cultural background important to you?

An excellent way of making an assessment of a potential practitioner is to arrange to have a brief chat on the phone: you could, for example, ask a few questions about the therapy and whether it could help for your or your child's health problem and take the opportunity to discuss fees and home visits; even a few minutes chat can give you a clue as to whether you could work with a practitioner. Advice from friends and colleagues can also be useful.

However, you might only be able to decide how you feel about a practitioner after a few sessions. It can be annoying, embarrassing and expensive to change practitioners once a course of treatment has actually begun, but if you have a problem you really want solved, and if you see healthcare as a long-term enterprise, it may be the best option.

Choosing a Suitable Therapy

Before it is possible to choose a therapy, you will first need to think about your aims, that is, what you hope to achieve from healthcare. For example:

1. Are you looking for something to help with poor sleep?
2. Is control of a secondary symptom, such as recurrent flu, your main concern?
3. Or are you wanting to focus on problems of mobility and muscle function, such as poor speech or walking?

As well as specific health problems, you might also want to consider what you want out of healthcare in general.

1. Are you looking for something you can use as self-help?
2. Do you want to learn a technique you could use on your child?
3. Or are you looking for a one-to-one relationship with a practitioner?

Once you have made this decision, you can use the information in Chapter 4 to start developing a list of therapies that you think could possibly help you achieve your goals. The next thing to decide is what is your first reaction towards each of the therapies you have listed. Do any therapies particularly attract you? Do you like the ideas behind one of the therapies or think you might enjoy some of the techniques involved? Choosing something that strikes a chord with you not only means you will enjoy treatment more but also increases your chances of success.

This does not mean, however, that you will inevitably find the most effective therapy, first time around. For reasons that are not entirely clear, there seems to be some kind of natural variation in how individuals respond to different therapies. It is not uncommon for someone to try a number of therapies before finding one that suits them best. Like finding the right practitioner, finding the right therapy can sometimes involve ending a course of treatment prematurely in order to start again somewhere else.

Other Issues in Choosing a Therapy and Practitioner

Though personal preference should always be the priority in making decisions about complementary medicine, there are a number of other issues and questions worth considering.

Different Therapies for Different Health Problems?

Despite what has been said about the importance of personal preference, it does seem that certain health problems are more amenable to treatment with some therapies than with others. For example, back pain is more usually associated with chiropractic than with herbal medicine. Listed below are suggested therapies for a number of health problems common in cerebral palsy and similar conditions. The recommendations should only be seen as a general pointer: you should read the rest of this chapter and the individual sections for each therapy in Chapter 4 before coming to any firm decisions.

You should remain aware of the fact that the listing of a therapy with certain health problems does not mean that that therapy will necessarily be of help; similarly, if a therapy is not listed, this does not mean that it cannot sometimes be effective at alleviating the symptoms in question.

Recurrent Infections Homoeopathy, herbal medicine and acupuncture can be helpful for a wide variety of infections. Aromatherapy is particularly useful in colds and flu, though benefit in bladder infections has also been reported. Dietary modification can also be effective for recurrent chest infections. Decreased susceptibility to infection has also been reported in a variety of other therapies, including osteopathy, shiatsu and reflexology.

Bowel and Bladder Problems For infections, see above. For constipation or diarrhoea, consider homoeopathy, herbal medicine, nutrition and reflexology. Massage and aroma-therapy can also be useful in the short term. Older children and adults might want to consider meditation and relaxation or yoga. For bedwetting and urinary incontinence, see homoeopathy, reflexology, acupuncture and shiatsu. For pain, see below.

Digestion and Appetite It appears that almost all complementary therapies improve digestion and appetite. However, see in particular herbal medicine and nutrition. For colic, see also homoeopathy, acupuncture and osteopathy.

Skin Problems See homoeopathy, herbal medicine and possibly nutrition. Aromatherapy is also said to be of help in certain skin conditions.

Pain It is difficult to generalize about pain in cerebral palsy and allied conditions as it can arise from so many different causes. For example, an appropriate therapy for pain caused by constipation may be inappropriate for pain caused by muscular spasm. That said, acupuncture is widely regarded to be an effective treatment for pain. Therapies such as massage, shiatsu, reflexology and healing can also be of benefit, particularly in the short term. In older children and adults, yoga and meditation/relaxation techniques are known to be highly effective means of pain relief.

Behaviour and Sleep Difficulties Many therapies can help soothe irritable and distracted children in the short term. (See massage and aromatherapy, healing, reflexology and shiatsu.) Osteopaths, chiropractors, acupuncturists and some homoeopaths say that they can effect more long-term change. For older children and adults with sleep difficulties, consider meditation and relaxation or shiatsu.

Speech Difficulties See 'Mobility and muscle function'.

Epilepsy It is very hard to make generalizations about epilepsy because its severity and response to treatment vary enormously. Therapies that have been reported to have been of benefit include acupuncture, cranial osteopathy and homoeopathy. Stress and anxiety can make seizures more likely in some people and so therapies such as shiatsu, aromatherapy and massage and healing may be of benefit, as might meditation or yoga for older adults and children.

Learning Disability The effects of complementary medicine on learning disability are discussed in detail on page 26. The therapies in which improvements in alertness and learning ability have been reported include acupuncture, osteopathy and homoeopathy. There have also been reports of benefit in healing and reflexology.

Mobility and Muscle Function See Chapter 2 (page 26) for a discussion of the effects of complementary medicine on mobility and muscle function. The main therapies reputed to have benefit are acupuncture and osteopathy. Spasm and involuntary movements are known to be exacerbated by stress and anxiety. So techniques such as aromatherapy and massage, reflexology, healing and shiatsu might have positive effects, although perhaps only in the short term. For older children and adults, yoga, tai chi and/or meditation techniques might be recommended. See also Alexander technique, Feldenkrais and Rolfing.

Families and Personal Preference

It is relatively easy for an adult seeking complementary medicine to interpret ideas about personal preference: he or she just chooses the therapy and practitioner thought to be most suitable and to have the greatest chance of success. With children, the situation can become more complicated. For a start, there is the problem of: whose personal preference? It is obvious that a very young child or baby will not be capable of making spoken decisions on healthcare; on the other hand, a teenager should surely be allowed some say in the decision-making process.

The general consensus among practitioners is that, though parents should make any final decisions, they should give as much weight as possible to the feelings of their child. Even babies can express their feelings towards a practitioner, and older children will often also be able to give some information as to whether they feel the therapy is helping. Both parent and child should be happy with the final choice of therapy and practitioner.

One immediate complication is that what children like, and what is good for them, may not always be identical. For example, take a child who enjoys aromatherapy massage – because it feels so nice – but dislikes acupuncture – because of the needles and because it can hurt sometimes. Is it not possible that acupuncture might well have tangible and lasting benefits for the child, benefits that might be lost if the parents decided on massage?

Another issue is what is known as resistance. It seems that a quite natural part of healthcare is for a person to adopt behaviours and attitudes that actually make healing more difficult. It is quite complicated to explain why this is so (see however, page 170) but one result of resistance is that a child may shy away from therapies and practitioners that can be of help.

A final problem is: what if parents disagree about a child's healthcare? Does it matter if they come to different decisions about which therapy and practitioner would be the best? Similarly, does it matter if one parent has no feelings one way or the other? The short answer is: yes, it usually does. The role of the family in healthcare is discussed in Chapter 5. One of the points made is that therapy seems to be most effective once the whole family becomes involved. It is clear that this will be a problem if there is significant disagreement on which course of action to take and so it is important for a family to come to some sort of consensus about healthcare plans.

Should I Choose a Practitioner Who Specializes in Treating Children?

A number of practitioners of complementary medicine specialize in the treatment of children. Some practitioners just happen to have a particular interest in treating children, and they have often built up considerable experience as a result. Others work almost exclusively with children and they may even describe themselves as 'paediatric osteopaths' or something similar.

Many parents are unsure of whether they should choose a practitioner purely on the basis that he or she specializes in treating children. There is no easy answer to this question. Obviously, all else being equal, it is generally an advantage to work with a practitioner who has had experience of similar cases, but is it really worth ignoring issues such as personal preference or travelling time?

Complementary therapy with children differs from that with adults in a number of ways. For a start, treatment is generally gentler and less invasive. For example, osteopaths rarely use a forceful manipulation on a child; similarly an acupuncturist will insert a needle for only a short period of time and an aromatherapist use only a few drops of essential oil. One of the reasons for this is that change may happen faster and more easily in children. For example, a period of time must pass before a homoeopath can tell whether a particular remedy has been effective or whether a different remedy should be tried. This period is generally shorter for children than for adults.

Another difference between the treatment of children and that of adults is that an adult will generally lie still on the treatment table if asked to. A child may fidget and move around, or even burst into tears if bored or hungry, and this is something that a practitioner can deal with more or less effectively. Finally, diagnosis is often more difficult with children: the practitioner may not be able to ask the child any direct questions or even ask how something feels during a session.

It is clear that a practitioner who is experienced in treating children will be better able to deal with these issues and concerns. On the other hand, you would clearly not be better off seeing a practitioner whom both you and your child distrusted, simply because of his or her special skills. As ever, it is up to every parent to decide what importance they give to a practitioner's particular specialism, and how much to their personality, cost and convenience.

Time and Money: How Long Will It Take and How Much Will It Cost?

In Chapter 2, it was pointed out that complementary medicine generally takes a longer time to achieve a result than orthodox medicine. However, it is often impossible to say exactly how much time a course of complementary therapy will take. Like orthodox medicine, complementary medicine does not always achieve its aims, and, if it doesn't work, the question of how long it takes to work becomes somewhat redundant.

The amount of time required for complementary medicine depends very much on the therapy concerned, and what its end goal will be. It is not hard to see why a course of acupuncture aiming to improve a child's mental and physical functioning will take longer than a course of homoeopathy for a minor infection.

An important concept in complementary medicine for people who have disabilities is that of 'management'. Many of the problems that disabled adults and children face result from a condition or process that is, in effect, permanent. For example, spasm is caused by damage to the nervous system, which is generally irreversible. Similarly, bowel problems and respiratory infections can be promoted by the use of a wheelchair, again, something that is unlikely to change. The idea of 'management' is that complementary therapies may be able to ameliorate some of the health problems associated with disability without removing them permanently. Regular 'top-up' treatments are then required to ensure that the symptoms do not return.

For example, Jeannie is a 4-year-old child who has an undiagnosed condition similar to cerebral palsy. Her problems are that she has sleep difficulties, recurrent chest infections and that she is often tense and irritable. Her parents took her to an aromatherapist, and they were pleased to find that she was generally calmer for a few days after treatment. Her chest infections were also less frequent. However, these two effects seemed dependent on continuing therapy: when aromatherapy was stopped for a few months, Jeannie gradually became more irritable and prone to infection.

The following figures are given as a general guide for two reasons: to give you some idea of what to expect from complementary medicine and so that you might be able to assess your progress once you start. They have not been given as a statement of fact as to what happens in complementary medicine.

It is clear that the cost of a course of complementary treatment can be high and this may place a significant financial burden on some individuals and families. In fact, a recent Scope report identified the high cost of treatment as the main obstacle to the greater use of complementary therapies by people with cerebral palsy. There are several ways to deal with this problem.

As part of developing a personal programme of healthcare (see below) you will have to assess how much time, money and effort you are willing to expend. This will often involve looking at your personal budget and/or that of your family. It is worth remembering that many people, particularly in the UK, see healthcare as a bit of an 'optional extra': perhaps this stems from the idea that we all

	Adults	**Children**
Average Length of 1 session	45 minutes–1 hour	20–40 minutes
Average cost of 1 session	£25. In some therapies, for example, homoeopathy, the first session is more expensive, perhaps £35–50. Expect to pay about an extra £5–10 if you are visited at home.	£15. More expensive for the first session in some therapies. There is a similar charge for outcalls.
Number of sessions before some change is seen	Practitioners say that some changes are normally noticed at least by the sixth session.	If changes are likely to occur at all, they normally do so by the fourth session.
How often should sessions be?	Sessions normally start weekly, going to fortnightly after a month or two, perhaps followed by quarterly or 6 weekly 'top-up' visits.	Sessions can be two or three times a week in the early stages. Gaps of more than three or four weeks can cause problems.
Length of a 'course' of treatment.	Some form of culmination is normally reached by sessions 12–15, though it may be at least two or three times that for serious or long-term problems such as those in cerebral palsy. Treatment often needs to be continuous. See also page 51.	As for adult. Regular treatment is sometimes needed for up to a year or more. See also page 51.

are somehow entitled to good health and that money used to that end is money that needn't be spent. Some authors have suggested that the cost of healthcare, and its benefits, should be compared with the cost and benefits of other parts of daily life, for example, an item of clothing, a car, a new stereo or a week's worth of beer and cigarettes.

There are a number of ways to cut the cost of therapy. Many schools of complementary medicine run clinics that offer treatment at a lower rate than normal, partly because some of each session will be devoted to the training of students. Healing is sometimes available in local community facilities for the price of a small donation, for those who can afford it. Complementary medicine is also often available at special schools and centres. For example, one school in London has a group of osteopaths who visit every week, and the regular teaching staff have received a basic training in massage.

One disadvantage of the two approaches outlined above is that it is unlikely that you will get to develop a relationship with a practitioner in a quiet and confidential atmosphere. In fact, where most clinics are concerned, it is common for a client to be treated by a different practitioner each time they visit.

There remain two other options: firstly, many practitioners have a sliding scale of fees and are happy to give treatment at a lower rate, if a normal charge would cause a client or family genuine hardship. Secondly, there are a number of sources of special funding for individuals encountering hardship and it is possible that such funds might be used for therapy. You will have to contact a social worker to help you put in an application for a grant.

However, perhaps the ultimate answer to the financial burden of complementary therapies is for them to be more widely available on the NHS. There may be a case for concerned parents and other individuals to put pressure on NHS institutions and staff to provide complementary therapies if they think that such therapies would meet an important health need.

Accessibility and Travel Time

Many of the places from which complementary practitioners work are not accessible to wheelchairs. One of the solutions is for practitioners to do 'outcalls', a visit to the client's home or place of work. However, it is not unusual for disabled people to have problems finding a practitioner who either has an accessible clinic or who is prepared to do an outcall. If this happens to you, it is worth challenging one of the inaccessible practitioners you have contacted and asking if he or she feels that disabled people should be excluded from treatment. Appealing to a practitioner's higher nature can work wonders.

Another issue is that of travelling time. It is becoming increasingly usual for people, especially parents, to travel many hundreds of miles to visit a practitioner, normally on the grounds that he or she is a renowned expert. There are a number of things worth saying about this practice. Firstly, complementary medicine normally takes a good number of regular treatments to become effective. People considering travelling long distances should think about the effect of doing so every week for 6 months. Secondly, travelling long distances requires time, money and effort that could be spent on other aspects of healthcare. Thirdly, there is evidence that treatment is less effective if it is associated with something unpleasant, such as a long journey. In short, travelling time should be seen as a serious consideration in deciding about complementary medicine.

Combining Therapies

The strengths and weaknesses of different therapies often lie in different areas. Therefore, when you are choosing a therapy, you should keep in mind the therapies that you, or your child, are using or intend to use. Chapter 4 should give you some idea of what each therapy is good at, and you can use this information to avoid combining similar techniques. For example, chiropractic and osteopathy have similar aims and methods and it is hard to think of a good reason to visit a chiropractor if you are already receiving osteopathy.

Another issue is that of the total number of different therapies worth combining. There are various reasons why, in complementary medicine at least, more does not always mean better.

1. If you are using a large number of different therapies, it becomes difficult to develop a strong relationship with any one practitioner.
2. It is hard for anyone to believe that each one of a large number of different therapies is being helpful.
3. Complementary practitioners say that the body's ability to respond to treatment is not infinite, and that beyond a certain amount of therapy a week, the body ceases to respond. A useful analogy can be found in sport: most people try to get fit using a limited number of sports, rather than by trying jogging, cycling, aerobics, swimming and rowing all at the same time.
4. Most disabled people have to deal with a large number of health professionals in the course of their lives. Restricting the number of complementary practitioners can help moderate problems such as lack of liaison between different professionals and the common feeling that there is little more to life than therapy.

Practical Issues

Unfortunately, you will probably not be able to make an entirely free choice of practitioner and therapy. For example, your choice might be limited by where you live, how much money you have, or, if transport or access is a problem, which practitioners are prepared to do outcalls. You might also find that certain practitioners are booked up and can take on no more clients.

You should not worry unduly about finding the perfect combination of practitioner and therapy. Many people have successful courses of treatment, despite coming across their practitioner quite by chance, and perhaps even being sceptical about their chance of success.

Getting Started

Once you have made a decision to visit a particular practitioner, there are various things you can do to ensure that healthcare progresses smoothly.

1. Make an appointment as soon as possible. It is not uncommon for people to decide what they want from healthcare, decide what they want to do about it, choose a therapy and practitioner, and then not do anything else for months or even years. To avoid this trap, take positive action as soon as you can.
2. Make a commitment for a fixed trial period. Some people try just one session of complementary medicine, observe no benefit and give up. Others take things one appointment at a time, deciding only to book more sessions if they experience benefit. These approaches can cause a number of problems. A good way of avoiding these is to book, and even pay for, somewhere between three and six appointments at a time.
3. Think about how you will assess your progress and plan for change. It is all too easy to drift through a course of treatment, without taking time to evaluate its benefit, or think about whether it would be worth changing things in some way. When you begin treatment, it is worth discussing the issue of evaluation with your practitioner. You could, for example, decide to re-evaluate your progress after a certain number of sessions.

Summary: How to Choose a Therapy and Practitioner

- Choosing a therapy and practitioner is more than just a case of avoiding quacks: it involves a positive decision about what you are looking for in healthcare.
- You will have to consider the other therapies you are using, a child's own preference of therapy and the role of the family. There is also the difficult issue of how to combine therapies.
- A useful way of putting all these problems and decisions together is to think about a *programme* of healthcare. Rather than seeing each therapy and practitioner as a separate part of a piecemeal pattern of care, a programme of healthcare involves each therapy being seen as part of a single enterprise.
- The most important point about a programme of healthcare is that it is planned and written down. Devising a programme of healthcare involves the following steps:
  - Decide what you want from healthcare.
  - Work out which therapies (both complementary and orthodox) could help you achieve your goals.
  - Choose which therapies you feel to be interesting or attractive, those that strike a chord with you.
  - Decide how much time and money you are willing and able to spend on achieving your goals.
  - Decide how to integrate different therapies, plus self-help, into a single programme of healthcare.
  - Find suitable practitioners.
  - Make a commitment to a fixed trial period.
  - Think about how you will assess your progress and make decisions to change if need be.
- More information on programmes of healthcare can be found in Chapter 5, which discusses liaison and co-operation between different health professionals.

Chapter 4

An Introduction to the Therapies

MASSAGE AND AROMATHERAPY

Introduction to Massage and Aromatherapy

Almost all cultures have developed and used systems of massage through the ages. In the West, the most prevalent form of massage in recent times has been what is known as Swedish massage. This traditionally focuses on the more physical aspects of treatment: massage is seen as a good way of promoting good general health by, for example, improving blood circulation, increasing muscle tone, easing joints and working on knots in connective tissue. Swedish massage also tends to be rather structured, with specific strokes used in set ways.

Recently, the more 'spiritual' aspects of massage – relaxation, calmness, wholeness – have been given a more central role. 'Holistic massage', one name for a modern form of massage, is more nurturing and comforting than the Swedish style. For example, a practitioner might gently hold and caress a part of the body and would make sure to avoid causing pain. Some practitioners also incorporate aspects of healing or shiatsu into their work.

Another recent innovation is the use of aromatherapy oils in treatment. These oils, which are known as 'essential oils', are distilled from plants and contain a concentrated mixture of the substances that give a plant its own particular aroma. Each different essential oil is believed to have a variety of healing properties.

Essential oils can have an effect on our emotions. Because some aromas are warm and soothing, whereas others are fresh and invigorating, a practitioner can use an essential oil to add to the calming or uplifting effect of a massage.

Some essential oils also have more specific properties. Scientific studies have demonstrated that many oils are active against bacteria, and a number have also been shown to have beneficial effects on fever, inflammation and pain. Aromatherapists have discovered many more properties by using traditional knowledge and experimentation. For example, various different oils are believed to be of benefit for mucus, intestinal gas, circulation and water retention.

Massage is a particularly effective way of using essential oils because as well as being breathed in, they can also be absorbed through the skin. Essential oils can also be used in a number of other ways. A popular 'self-help' method is to add a few drops of oil to a bath. Alternatively, oils may be used in compresses or inhalations. Essential oils can also be vaporized in a special burner, so that their smell and therapeutic effect fills a whole room.

Massage and aromatherapy are popular techniques and their use in hospitals, special schools and other institutions is growing rapidly. There have, however, been two major barriers to their wider acceptance: lax standards of training and qualification, an issue that is dealt with in the section 'Massage and aromatherapy in practice' below, and the association, in the West, between touch and sex. This particular problem has been exacerbated by the fact that some advertisements for 'massage' are merely fronts for prostitution. The result is that many people feel uncomfortable with the whole idea of professional massage. It is worth pointing out, however, that reputable massage practitioners have a good understanding of the therapeutic use of touch: in practice, many of the anxieties that some people have about feeling uncomfortable, or sexual, during a massage are quickly diffused by the strong, sure and directed touch of the practitioner.

That said, there are occasions when it is worth discussing these matters with a practitioner. For example, one parent of an adolescent who had a learning disability expressed some concern over the possible sexual implications of massage. As a result, the practitioner made sure to explain the purpose of the work to the client beforehand and to modify the massage in an appropriate way.

Visiting a Practitioner of Massage and Aromatherapy

Practitioners of massage and aromatherapy work from warm, quiet rooms. The practitioner will take a short case history and perhaps offer the client a choice of different oils to use. The initial chat is also a good opportunity for you to state any preferences you might have for the form of the massage. You might prefer it to be energetic and invigorating for instance, or perhaps more calming and soothing. You might also wish to mention any areas you would like particular attention paid to, for example, a sore back or cold feet.

Massage normally takes place on a special treatment couch. The client will be asked to undress, with privacy maintained by the use of towels. The practitioner will use an oil, to which a few drops of essential oils may have been added, to help the hands move over the surface of the skin. A full body massage can last anywhere between 45 minutes and an hour-and-a-half for an adult – about a third of that time for a child – after which the practitioner will often leave you to rest for a short while.

This is not a set form however: massage can often just consist of a good back rub sitting up in a room with other people. Most practitioners are fairly adaptable and if removing clothes or using a massage table is something that would cause discomfort or uncertainty there should be no inconvenience in arranging some suitable position to work in. Some sessions consist of a gentle kneading and rubbing through clothes, particularly when a practitioner does an outcall.

With young children, undressing and working on a massage couch rarely presents any difficulties. Children often relax and fall asleep during treatment; others will stay awake quite calmly, obviously enjoying the feelings of being rubbed and squeezed. If a child does get upset or restless, the practitioner may be able to work on the head, hands, back or feet while the child is cradled in a parent's arms.

One of the most positive aspects of massage and aromatherapy is that it can be used by parents themselves. The practitioner may demonstrate some simple massage strokes to be practised at home, and they might also make up an aromatherapy oil that can be used for massage, added to a bath or used in a burner. Many parents enjoy becoming actively involved in treatment in this way and it can be of benefit to children to receive regular treatment, especially as essential oils may not stay in the body for long periods.

Massage and Aromatherapy Treatment

General Issues

Relaxation is one of the most well-known and important benefits of massage:

> The treatment is just so relaxing. It relieves all the tension in my back, neck and shoulders. I feel very calm and soothed afterwards.

Massage brings about relaxation in a number of different ways. Firstly, the act of lying still and concentrating on the practitioner's touch can be deeply relaxing. Massage also feels good, and it takes place in a warm and comforting environment.

A practitioner may also attempt to bring about relaxation in a more directed fashion. Many massage strokes aim to release tension held in muscles; another common technique is to apply light pressure to the chest or back in rhythm with the breathing. A practitioner trained in aromatherapy may choose oils that have sedative properties.

Improved sleep is a common result of massage and aromatherapy treatment. Sometimes, a client will drift off to sleep during the session. Another common experience is to find that the night's sleep after the massage was especially deep and restful:

> I hadn't really slept for two weeks since the injury, but about five minutes into the massage, I was out like a light.

> Zorina has had far fewer restless nights since she has been receiving massage. Sometimes, when it does look as though she might have trouble getting off, I massage her back with the oil the aromatherapist gave us.

Aromatherapy oils can also be placed in a burner, so that their smell fills the entire room at bedtime.

One general benefit of massage, which has received considerable attention, is that of improvement in self-image. This term can be used in two separate ways. Firstly, self-image can refer to an individual's general feelings about themselves and their body. Taken in this sense, self-image is somewhat similar to self-esteem. In Chapter 2 it was pointed out that some disabled people have problems with the image they have of their own body: they may see themselves as ugly or deformed or as somehow unworthy.

Massage can help mitigate these feelings in a number of ways. The act of being touched, in a caring and nurturing manner, can of itself improve self-image. Moreover, the pleasure and relaxation that results from massage may lead to the realization that the body can be a source of feelings of well-being, as well as those of frustration and pain (see also page 19).

Self-image can also be used in the sense of awareness of the body. Some people report a general feeling of being in touch with themselves after massage, others experience more specific improvements in their perception of posture, position and movements.

> When I was being massaged, it felt like a stroke up my back was traversing three countries. Massage made me aware of the splits and divisions in me. I certainly gain self-acceptance through touch.

Improved awareness of the body can have important consequences for physical function. It is worth pointing out, however, that there are a number of techniques that are specifically designed to improve body awareness and which might be seen as more effective than massage at achieving this end. See the Alexander technique (page 110) and Feldenkrais (page 113).

Physical Benefits

A number of the more tangible benefits of massage and aromatherapy derive from the relaxation that treatment so often affords. For example, as was pointed out in Chapter 3, stress and anxiety can promote spasticity and involuntary movements. At least part of the short-term improvements in muscle tone and mobility that can result from massage may be attributed to the effects of relaxation.

> I used mainly lavender and camomile oils blended for an all over massage for Philip. I found it really helped relax his "jerky" muscle spasms and relaxed him.

However, massage may have more direct effects on the physical body and this is why physiotherapists use massage as part of their work. Massage treatment involves kneading and manipulating muscles and this may ease tension, cramp and stiffness and improve blood circulation:

> After a massage, you can see that Sam's hands have opened out and relaxed.

> Anne's hands and feet are normally ice cold, but they feel soft and warm after a treatment session.

> Massage relieves all the pain and stiffness in my neck and shoulders. It feels great for a couple of days after the session.

By increasing flexibility and blood flow, massage may sometimes lead to improvements in mobility. In some settings, the dual use of physiotherapy and massage has facilitated this process:

> The staff [introduced] physiotherapy exercises as her limbs became warm and supple from the massage. Regular massage increased the flexibility in her hips and back so that she could stand straighter and walk using more of her own balance and weight.

Spasm may also be affected by massage. It is known, for example, that stretching a muscle in a certain way can help relieve spasm. One problem is that whereas a physiotherapist will generally have the training and experience to reduce spasm in a muscle, it is unlikely that many complementary massage practitioners possess the specialist skills required to bring about a specific change of this nature. Similarly, though the prevention of pressure sores and contractures may be helped by a complementary massage practitioner, such an individual will not be as well placed as a physiotherapist to assess and treat such problems.

One area in which many practitioners have provided a useful service, however, is in the treatment of problems of the digestive tract such as indigestion and constipation.

Massage on the lower back and abdomen and gentle strokes on the stomach are said to be helpful:

> Alan ... becomes constipated and often became very bad tempered after lunch at the day centre. Staff ... started to massage his abdomen regularly. He started to go to the toilet more regularly and became less distressed after lunch.

Some parents who have learned a few simple massage strokes for the stomach have said that this has been an enormous help for their child's constipation.

Essential oils may be prescribed to enhance the physical effects of massage. Black pepper, for example, is a rubefacient, which means that it increases blood circulation. So an aromatherapist who considered that increased blood flow would serve a useful purpose might add a measured few drops of the essential oil of black pepper to the massage oil.

A number of essential oils are said to be anti-spasmodic. The reason why peppermint is useful for indigestion is that peppermint oil relieves spasm in the intestines. However, it is not really known whether essential oils can have anti-spasmodic effects on skeletal muscles (such as those in the arm or leg).

A particularly important use of aromatherapy is in the treatment and control of infection. Aromatherapists have made a number of claims about the control of infection. They say that:

1. Essential oils can strengthen the immune system.
2. Essential oils can fight bacteria directly, a claim that is supported by a number of scientific studies.
3. Essential oils can relieve some of the symptoms of infection, for example, cedar leaf oil is a decongestant and is therefore useful for respiratory infections.

These statements are supported by the experience of clients of aromatherapy, particularly children. Improved resistance to infection is the benefit most commonly reported by parents:

He never has recurring chest infections, which would ordinarily be the case in his condition. He is extremely healthy and energetic.

A number of the mothers at the centre have commented that, since the aromatherapist started work here, the number of respiratory infections that the children get has reduced to a more normal level.

For more on aromatherapy for recurrent infections, see under herbal medicine on page 132.

Behaviour and Social Skills

One of the results of massage and aromatherapy can be improved behaviour and social skills. Again, relaxation plays a significant role in bringing about such improvements: many behaviours are promoted by tension and anxiety, and by agitation and excitement.

Massage and aromatherapy are often used to soothe irritable and distracted children. A full body massage can sometimes send a child off to sleep, but even a gentle hand or foot rub can be helpful in calming a child and diffusing tension.

In those with learning disabilities, relaxation training has been shown to reduce disruptive behaviours (see page 116) and workers who have used massage have noticed similar effects:

Denise has inexplicable outbursts of temper and violence towards objects. She can be very excitable, but through massage becomes much quieter and calmer. There is benefit for her in just keeping still in a relaxed way.

One of the most interesting and important areas in which massage has been found to be of benefit is in cases of self-harm:

Jean was continually thrashing backwards and forwards, punching her head with her fists, slapping her head and face.

... The aromatherapist spent two hours with her using a massage oil made up with relaxing essential oils. At first any contact with Jean was met with total rejection ... [but] during the last half hour ... Jean appeared relaxed and was lying back in the bean bag, with her hands behind her head, smiling and sometimes laughing.

Massage is believed to be helpful in cases of self-harm because rubbing the skin releases a class of substances known as endorphins. These dampen down the perception of pain, something that explains why massage can be helpful for painful conditions. It is thought that self-injurious behaviour stimulates the production of endorphins and that people who self-harm are 'addicted' to the feelings that are produced in this way. Massage may provide someone who self-harms an alternative way of eliciting these sensations.

Massage and aromatherapy involve touch and, as such, they can be a useful means of stimulating communication and interaction, especially for those who have sensory disabilities. A number of workers have used massage to develop relationships with individuals who had previously been unresponsive to human contact. Touch can be a way of 'getting to know' someone and there have been reports of individuals whose first significant attempts at communication and relationships resulted from massage. Massage can also be used to overcome the 'tactile defensiveness' that is found in many people who have learning disabilities, and that can inhibit learning and other tasks.

Another interesting application of massage and aromatherapy is in what is known as 'multisensory massage'. One practitioner defines this as 'the use of different textures, tools, talcs, lotions and [aromatherapy] oils ... to provide stimulation to the senses'. Multisensory massage has a number of different aims. One of the most important is to impart the information that there is an outside world, and that it can be stimulating. Another is to improve general awareness of tactile experiences, to demonstrate the existence, and individual characteristics, of different objects.

Both of these aims are important because people with learning disabilities may fail to reach out and explore their environment as a result of physical and sensory disabilities, something that may be compounded by the unstimulating surroundings found in institutions. More information on the use of massage and aromatherapy for communication and stimulation with those with learning difficulties can be found in a book called *Aromatherapy and Massage for People with Learning Difficulties* (see Further Reading.)

Massage and Aromatherapy in Practice

Massage and aromatherapy are often seen as separate disciplines. Certainly most practitioners identify themselves with one rather than both therapies, and there are separate registers for each.

Finding a reputable practitioner of massage or aromatherapy presents a number of problems. Firstly, there is no single, widely accepted register for either therapy. Secondly, particularly in the case of massage, the link between a practitioner's qualifications and his or her ability is much weaker than in many other therapies. Thirdly, and worst of all, massage is sometimes used as a front for prostitution: some people who advertise massage are not therapeutic masseurs.

A further complication is that many otherwise fully competent massage practitioners may learn a bit of basic aromatherapy and will occasionally mix together some nice smelling oils when the mood takes them. Though this is obviously somewhat different from the use of specific essential oils for a specific therapeutic purpose, it can sometimes be difficult for a member of the public to know exactly what they are getting.

There are some registers of massage and aromatherapy, and these can sometimes provide a useful resource. Many of the registers are associated with a particular school and primarily list its graduates. Given that this inevitably leads to a large and confusing array of different registers, the British Register of Complementary Practitioners (see page 178) can be of help. There is a list for both massage and aromatherapy and two grades of competence are listed for each.

It is worth pointing out that large numbers of massage and aromatherapy practitioners are not affiliated to any registering body. Advice on unregistered practitioners is given in Chapter 3. Many unregistered practitioners advertise as 'ITEC Qualified'. ITEC is a rather basic course that includes Swedish massage and elementary physiology and anatomy. Some people take ITEC as part of a longer and more thorough course, but there are those who take classes purely to get through the exam.

It may be advisable to check that any practitioner located through a register or a personal recommendation is competent to practise. Chapter 3 (page 38) contains some useful advice on this subject. However, it is important to remember the central importance of personal preference. A brief chat on the phone can often be a help. It can be a good idea to ask about the style of massage they practise (Holistic? Swedish? Vigorous? More soothing?) Have they had any experience working with children? It can also be a good idea to try just one massage with a practitioner to see how you get on: if you (or your child) don't enjoy it or feel better for it, it would probably be a good idea to look elsewhere.

Massage and Aromatherapy: a Summary

- Massage is the manipulation of the soft tissues of the body, such as the muscles, for therapeutic purposes. Aromatherapy is the use of aromatic oils extracted from plants and is often used together with massage.
- Massage and aromatherapy are extremely relaxing. They can calm irritable and distracted children and improve sleep.

- Some disabled people who have received massage say that the touch leads to a better self-image and greater self-acceptance.
- The physical benefits of massage and aromatherapy can include relieving stiffness and tension, improving blood flow and easing constipation. Such effects are usually short term.
- A number of individuals have reported experiencing fewer colds and flu after aromatherapy treatment.
- In those with learning disabilities, massage has helped reduce disruptive behaviours. It has also been used to foster communication.

Resources

Send SAEs to:

London and Counties Society of Physiologists
330 Lytham Road
Blackpool FY4 1DW
Tel: 0253 408443

Massage Therapy Institute of Great Britain
Tel: 081 208 1607

Association of Massage Practitioners
Contact through:
The Dancing Dragon School
115 Manor Road
London N16 5PB
Tel: 071 275 8002

London School of Sports Massage
88 Cambridge Street
London SW1V 4QG
Tel: 071 834 1849

The British Register of Complementary Practitioners
PO Box 194
London SE16 1QZ (enclose a large SAE)

Aromatherapy Organizations Council
3 Latymer Close
Braybrooke
Market Harborough
Leicestershire LE16 8LN
Tel: 0455 615446

Register of Qualified Aromatherapists
52 Barrack Lane
Aldwick
Bognor Regis
West Sussex PO21 4DD
Tel: 0243 262035

International Society of Professional Aromatherapists
Hinckley and District Hospital and Health Centre
The Annex
Mount Road
Hinckley
Leicestershire LE10 1AG
Tel: 0455 637987

International Federation of Aromatherapists
4 Eastmearn Road
London SE21 8HA
Tel: 081 846 8066

REFLEXOLOGY

Introduction to Reflexology

Reflexology is a special type of massage in which certain areas of the foot are believed to correspond to the organs or structures of the body. Damage or disease in an organ is reflected in the corresponding area, or reflex zone, of the

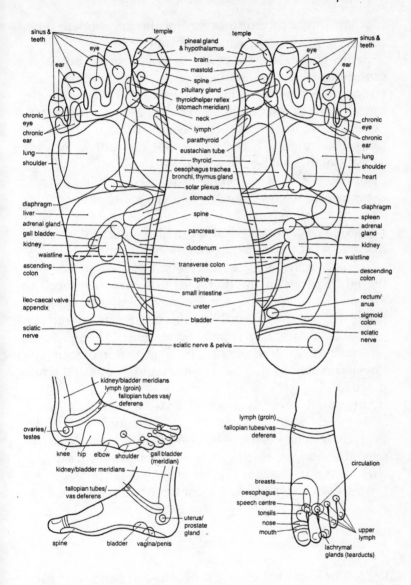

Figure 1. A reflexology map of the feet showing zones and corresponding areas of the body.

foot, and by a careful massage of the appropriate reflex zone, the practitioner can help promote healing.

Reflexologists evaluate a person's state of health by observing the feet. The bony structure, the colour and temperature, the condition of the skin and the tone of the muscles are all seen to give important information. Practitioners also assess the state of each reflex zone by gentle use of the fingers. If the reflex zone is healthy, the only sensation that will be felt is pressure. If there is some disorder, however, a feeling of pain or pricking may be experienced. Such a disorder might be merely due to some immediate strain (such as will be felt in the eyes after a day working at a computer) but it can also indicate damage or disease, whether medically diagnosed or not.

Though reflexology sounds somewhat unusual, and though it is one of the therapies that is most difficult to explain from a Western scientific viewpoint, it enjoys great popularity amongst rehabilitation professionals such as physiotherapists, nurses and occupational therapists. In fact, reflexology is recognized by the Chartered Society of Physiotherapy as falling within regular physiotherapy practise.

One of reflexology's major advantages in disability work is that it does not require any special equipment. Moreover, there is no need for the client to undress or to lie in a special position: if need be, a client can be treated in a wheelchair. It is thus easy for practitioners to make outcalls, and proceed with therapy with a minimum of difficulty.

Visiting a Practitioner of Reflexology

Reflexologists usually reserve the first appointment for a general case history and a thorough examination of the feet. Treatment normally starts with the second session: the practitioner will work on the reflex zones assessed as being disordered and attempt to bring them back towards a more normal state by a gentle set of massages.

Reflexology treatment is generally very relaxing and calming. As the practitioner works on the feet, he or she asks the client if any painful sensations are being experienced. The pain is not severe and feels quite unlike that which you might experience after an injury or joint problem; it may even be accompanied by a sense of well-being, somewhat like having a sore muscle massaged.

Feedback from the client about areas that feel painful can help the practitioner diagnose and treat. However, this information is not essential, and accomplished practitioners do not generally have significant problems with young children or with people who have impaired sensation in their feet.

It is common for clients to experience diarrhoea, sweating or increased passage of urine in the first few days and weeks after starting reflexology. Practitioners put this down to increased activity of the elimination systems of the body and see such side-effects as a positive sign. Similar changes may take place during treatment. Some people find that they start to sweat in a session; others, however, feel shivery or cold: this is a sign of over-stimulation and indicates that treatment should be stopped.

Reflexology Treatment

Non-specific Effects of Reflexology

One of the most immediate benefits of reflexology is deep relaxation:

> When I have reflexology, my body feels nice and relaxed. This will last for a few days.

Such relaxation can often be of great importance to children with behavioural difficulties. A particularly dramatic case is given by a physiotherapist who uses reflexology in her everyday hospital work:

The baby had cried and screamed since birth and the mother was understandably upset and exhausted. The child quietened down almost as soon as I started treatment and was fast asleep by the end of the session.

Though the effects of reflexology are rarely as immediate, many parents have found that their children are generally less irritable after a course of treatment. Reflexology has been reported to improve sleep and this may also be due to its relaxing effects. A common experience is that sleep is particularly deep after a treatment session, and that sleep patterns gradually improve over time.

Two other reported non-specific benefits of reflexology have much in common with the effects of other complementary therapies. Firstly, many people have noticed that they or their children experience fewer bouts of colds and flu after reflexology:

The treatment seems to clear up snotty noses.

Secondly, many also notice an increase in general wellbeing:

I feel stronger in myself and more energetic.

Specific Effects of Reflexology Treatment

One benefit commonly reported by people with cerebral palsy who have experienced reflexology is an improvement in muscle tone. Improvements in spasticity, spasm and involuntary movements are often marked, and this may lead to improvement in function, particularly speech:

I have spasms and I am stiff. I can't walk without help. With the reflexology, the stiffness improved and the spasms decreased. My walking got better. So did my speech and breathing, and even my GP commented on that.

After a session, I can walk better and I can straighten my knees.

Richenda is much easier to handle in bed: her body isn't spasming so much.

Unfortunately, these effects do not appear to be long-lasting, particularly in adults. Typical comments include: 'If I go without treatment for 3 or 4 weeks I slip back' and 'I am so much better after a treatment but the effects only last a few days.' The first of the comments above was made by a man who received all fifteen of his reflexology treatments over a 3-month period. He now says: 'I'm back the way I was before; none of the effects has been long-term.' This problem is not uncommon in complementary medicine and is discussed further in Chapter 5 (page 168).

One reputed benefit of reflexology, however, does seem to be longer lasting:

The treatment perked her up. Before my daughter was all tired and floppy. You'd have to keep waking her up at school and she didn't move her arms or legs much. After the course of treatment, she was much more awake and alert and she has stayed that way ever since.

A physiotherapist who uses reflexology at a special school has made a similar observation:

The children become more aware in general. From being withdrawn and unresponsive they become more curious.

This effect seems most marked in younger children: there do not seem to be analogous case histories in adults. The effects of reflexology treatment for people with cerebral palsy and allied conditions appear somewhat similar to the effects of shiatsu (page 96 for more information).

Reflexology in Practice

The competence of practitioners of reflexology varies widely in the UK. Institutions professing to teach reflexology also vary in their methods and standards and there is a plurality of professional bodies, each generally associated with a single school and registering only graduates of that school. The accreditation of reflexology practitioners is in a chaotic state and represents much of what is worst about complementary medicine.

On the plus side, the British School of Reflex Zone Therapy of the Feet (BSRZTF) is an excellent organization that has done much to ensure high standards of practice and promote the use of reflexology within orthodox medicine. The school only trains those with medical or paramedical qualifications, the majority of the intake being registered nurses, physiotherapists and occupational therapists. The disadvantage of the BSRZTF is that its members tend to have busy professional lives that restrict private practice and this can limit opportunities for new clients. The Association of Chartered Physiotherapists in Reflex Therapy (ACPORT) is also probably a safe bet.

Two other useful organizations include the Association of Reflexologists, which is one of the few organizations that was not set up for the sole purpose of accrediting graduates from an associated school, and the British Reflexology Association, which registers individuals who have completed a course of study at the Bayley School of Reflexology, one of the oldest and most well-established schools. It is also worth noting that there is also a reflexology division of the British Register of Complementary Practitioners.

In conclusion, you have three choices if you are seeking a competent practitioner of reflexology: you can contact the BSRZTF or ACPORT or you can use one of the other organizations to locate a practitioner and then make sure for yourself that the person you are referred to is competent to practise. The section in Chapter 3 contains some useful advice on this subject.

Reflexology: a Summary

- Reflexology is a type of massage in which areas of the foot are believed to correspond to other parts of the body.
- It is deeply relaxing and has been used to calm irritable children.
- It has been reported that reflexology can improve muscle tone, sometimes leading to improved function. However, this does seem to be a short-term effect.
- Reflexology is reputed to improve alertness in some children.

Resources

Send SAEs to:

British School of Reflex Zone Therapy of the Feet
87 Oakington Avenue
Wembley Park
London HA9 8HY
Tel: 081 908 2201

The Association of Chartered Physiotherapists in Reflex Therapy
7 Waggon Road
Hadley Wood
Herts EN4 0PU

Association of Reflexologists
27 Old Gloucester Street
London WC1 3XX
Tel: 071 237 6523

British Reflexology Association
Monks Orchard
Whitbourne
Hereford and Worcester WR6 5RB
Tel: 0886 21207

British Register of Complementary Practitioners
PO Box 194
London SE16 1QZ (enclose a large SAE)

HEALING

Introduction to Healing

Healing is more widely known as 'spiritual' or 'faith' healing. It is normally associated with the activities of the populist church. The reason why the more general term is used here is that, contrary to popular belief, most healing does not take place within a religious context. Neither does it require faith: in the United States, for example, many nurses use a form of healing as part of their every-day hospital work.

The common belief of all healers is that a human being can induce healing solely by an effort of will. The details vary, but a common idea is that healing energy exists all around us and that the healer can channel this energy to the person in need. This is often done through the hands, with the healer placing the palms of his or her hands on or near the person being healed. The majority of healers say that they can sense energy around a person and that where they place their hands depends on whether this energy is depleted or in excess in different parts of the body. Some healers try to assess and correct the energy at specific places, which they call 'centres' or 'chakras'; others are more concerned with the state of energy in general.

However, it is important to remember that you do not have to share your healer's beliefs about healing, or about spirituality. A good healer will neither demand or expect that you conform to his or her personal faith: in fact, it is quite possible to have a course of healing without ever knowing what your healer's personal faith might be.

One of the advantages of healing is that it can be used in addition to any other therapy, conventional or otherwise. It is particularly worth looking at if you are unsure of what you want from complementary healthcare or if you are trying therapies that do not concentrate on relaxation, for example, homoeopathy.

Visiting a Healer

Healers work in a variety of contexts: at a client's home, at the practitioner's place of work, at a healing centre or even in a hospital. Some healers like to talk before healing, especially in the first session; others work entirely by intuition.

A healing session typically lasts between 15 minutes and an hour. The client usually sits upright in a chair, though healing can be done lying down. It is unnecessary to remove any clothes. The practitioner places their hands on and near the surface of the skin and concentrates on moving energy in an appropriate way.

Healing is very soothing and calming, but at the same time, many people feel quite invigorated after a session. It is also common to experience sensations such as heat, coolness or tingling and these can get quite intense. Some people have a direct feeling of energy moving through their body.

Children tend to get very sleepy during healing. Even if they have been over-active and irritable, they may quickly settle down and relax once the healing session begins.

It can take a little time to come back to reality after healing, so healers often suggest a short lie down and rest. Many healers use this time to talk as many people find it easier to communicate when they are calm and relaxed. Some healers lay great emphasis on the counselling element of healing: in the US, some professional nurses practise healing in a form known as 'therapeutic touch' and they often use healing specifically to help patients put feelings into words. Some healers use the time after a session to advise on relaxation or visualization exercises to use at home (see page 115).

Healing for Disabled People

One of the popular misconceptions of healing is that it is all about 'miracle cures'. From a disabled person or carer's point of view, it is very unfortunate that this has become epitomized by the empty wheelchair or the no-longer-needed crutch held aloft.

It is true that there have been cases where individuals have made dramatic progress after healing. One example that has gained considerable media attention is that of a boy who has cerebral palsy and who improved from almost zero mobility and alertness to a state where he uses only a single crutch for walking and attends a normal school. It is worth making several points. Firstly, as was explained in Chapter 2 (page 27), it is often difficult to tell what contribution any particular therapy makes to an individual's progress. Secondly, it is often difficult to tell how an individual might have progressed without therapy: there are many cases where children have made 'remarkable progress' and this is not always attributable to any particular therapeutic intervention.

Finally, but most importantly, cases where individuals make dramatic progress are exceptional, and do not reflect the general experience of individuals and families who use healing. As has already been pointed out, looking for 'miracles' can often blind people to the more everyday benefits that complementary medicine can sometimes afford.

The most common remark that parents make about healing, is that it has calmed and soothed their children:

> He's very relaxed and sleepy during the treatment, even if he's been haring around beforehand. The calmness normally lasts the rest of the day.

> The first improvement was that she started sleeping through the night after a healing session. After a while, she started sleeping better through the other nights of the week as well.

The second comment is interesting in that it reflects a common experience of complementary therapy. At first, the relaxing and calming effects of treatment may last for the duration of the session, or perhaps for a few hours afterwards. However, after a number of treatments, the changes may become longer lasting. In some cases, the improved mood and behaviour last a few days; in others, they last until the next weekly or fortnightly treatment session. In a few cases, they become effectively permanent:

> She is much less tense and irritable than she used to be.

One of the most important and beneficial effects of relaxation is that, in some cases at least, it can result in reduced frequency of epileptic seizures. Though a number of healers have reported cases where this has occurred, it must be said that it is not really known how healing might affect epilepsy.

Relaxation might also be of benefit for mobility. This is because anxiety and tension can promote spasticity and involuntary movements. However, again, little is known about the effects of healing on muscle tone and movement.

The other major benefit noticed by parents is improved motivation and confidence. A parent may say that a child seems generally happier and less tense, and that his or her personality is now more apparent:

> He is much more confident nowadays and I'm sure that this has been part of the reason why his speech has improved so much.

> She is much happier to do things for herself.

The experiences of adults who try healing are not dissimilar to those of children. Again, the two most prominently noticed effects are relaxation and improved mood and motivation. One of the interesting ways in which some people notice this improvement in mood is that though a problem may still be there, it doesn't bother them so much:

> Healing has given me such calm and peace. The spasm and pain are still there, but I just don't seem to notice them so much.

Healing in Practice

Healers are represented by various organizations. The National Federation of Spiritual Healers (NFSH) is the largest in the UK and it does not promote any particular religious viewpoint. As a member of the Confederation of Healing Organizations, their healers work to a strict code of ethics. The NFSH also provides an excellent contact and referral service and so there is no doubt that they should be the first point of contact for anyone interested in healing.

It is possible, of course, that you might have a particular reason to go elsewhere, for example, if you wanted a healer of a particular religious denomination. If you are unsure where to look, contact the Confederation of Healing Organizations.

You can also get healing in a group setting. Often a local group will take over a room or a hall for an evening and you can get healing there. Some of these places have a wonderful atmosphere and some people find it a more comfortable context than a one-to-one session. The down side is that you might not get to build up a relationship with a practitioner, that talking is difficult and that you might get only a short session of healing. Also, some of the centres are not wheelchair accessible. You can get details of healing centres from the NFSH.

Finally, if money is a problem, it is worth knowing that many healers do not charge for their services, asking only for a donation of what you can afford.

Healing: a Summary

- Healers believe that they can induce healing purely by an effort of will. The technique need not be associated with particular religious viewpoints.
- Healing is extremely relaxing. It has been reported to improve sleep and behaviour in some children.
- Many people who receive healing say that it improves their mood, motivation and general sense of well-being.

Resources

National Federation of Spiritual Healers
Old Manor Farm Studio
Sunbury-on-Thames
Middx TW16 6RG
Tel: 0932 783164

Send a request 'to be referred to a registered spiritual healer in my area' with a SAE.

Wilfred A Watts
Secretary
Confederation of Healing Organisations
25 Ducane Court
London
SW17 7JQ

Send SAE for details of other healing organizations.

Caring and Sharing Trust
Cotton's Farmhouse
Whiston Road
Cogenhoe
Northamptonshire NN7 1NK
Tel: 0604 891487

A healing centre specializing in treating disabled children.

THE METAMORPHIC TECHNIQUE AND POLARITY

Two therapies that show marked similarities to healing are the metamorphic technique and polarity. Though each has developed an autonomous set of practices and beliefs, the experiences and effects of treatment are very much like those of healing.

In polarity therapy, the practitioner places hands on the client's body in a systematic way, aiming to diagnose and treat blocks in energy flow. The originator of polarity therapy, Dr Randolph Stone, was originally an osteopath and naturopath and so both gentle manipulation and dietary advice also form part of polarity work.

The metamorphic technique involves a gentle massage up and down the insides of the feet and corresponding areas on the head and hands. The practitioner uses gentle, intuitive stroking motions and there may be some work just off the surface of the skin.

Metamorphic technique is very easy to learn and it is common that, after a few visits to a practitioner, a family will be taught the technique to use with each other. This emphasis on self-help, and the awareness of the importance of family involvement, must be seen as one of the most positive aspects of the metamorphic technique.

The governing body of the metamorphic technique, the Metamorphic Association, has a high degree of disability awareness: it has been particularly active in making the technique available at day centres, rehabilitation units and other institutions (where the response from the clients and staff has generally been very positive) and it has also fostered debate on work with people who have learning disabilities.

Resources

For lists of practitioners, send SAEs to:

Metamorphic Association
67 Ritherdon Road
London SW17 8QE
Tel: 081 672 5951

British Polarity Council
5 Bullkamore Court
South Brent
Devon TQ10 9LQ
Tel: 0364 42143

ORIENTAL MEDICINE

ACUPUNCTURE

Introduction to Acupuncture

Acupuncture is the most well-known technique of traditional Chinese medicine, a system that also incorporates herbalism, massage, diet and exercise. The technique involves the insertion of extremely fine needles through the skin at special points; this is thought to balance the body's energy and stimulate healing.

The principles of traditional Chinese medicine are quite complex and can be difficult for a Westerner to grasp. The workings of the human body are seen to be controlled by a

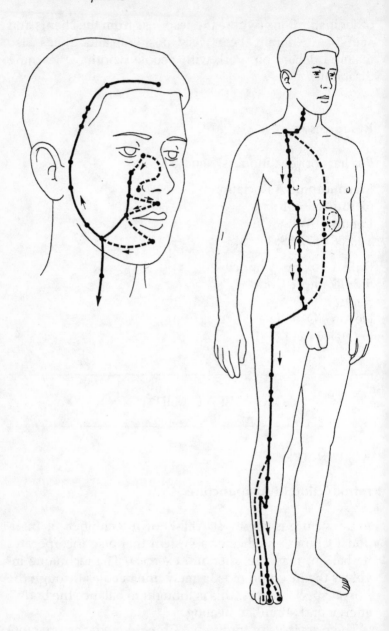

Figure 2. The stomach meridian showing acupuncture points.

vital force or energy called *chi*, which circulates between the organs along set channels called meridians. There are twelve meridians, each of which corresponds to the major functions or organs of the body such as the lungs or bladder, and *chi* energy must flow in the correct strength and quality through each of these meridians for health to be maintained.

Energy imbalances (which are associated with illness) can be corrected by a number of means; in acupuncture, needles are placed at special points on the meridians, and depending on how the needle is manipulated (for example, it may be gently twirled in place) the energy is either drawn to the meridian or dispersed from it. Herbs, diet and exercise can also be used to modify the energy state of the meridians.

Acupuncture is one of the most highly regarded complementary therapies. Large numbers of scientific studies have demonstrated its effectiveness and many doctors and physiotherapists practise acupuncture either exclusively, or in addition to conventional medicine.

Visiting an Acupuncturist

Most traditional acupuncture practitioners work from private practices that provide a comfortable place to sit and a treatment couch. In the first session, the practitioner takes a full case history, asking questions about lifestyle, diet, work and medical history. The practitioner will also make observations of the colour and quality of the skin and tongue and use a 'pulse diagnosis', a special technique whereby the energy of the meridians may be assessed by feeling the strength, rhythm and quality of the pulse.

Needles will often not be used until the second session. On average, between two and six needles are inserted through the skin. They are left in place for on average about half an hour or so (less for children), and during this time they may be gently manipulated by the practitioner.

As the needles are very fine – not much thicker than a human hair – they do not cause pain in the same way as injections; in fact, it is possible to remain unaware that a needle has been inserted. If the needle is correctly placed at an acupuncture point, there is a slight feeling of heaviness or distension. Once they have overcome their initial nervousness, most people find that acupuncture is very relaxing and leaves them feeling quite 'up' and invigorated after treatment.

Practitioners of acupuncture also use a technique called moxibustion, which is the burning of a special herb (moxa) on, or just above, the surface of the skin. This is thought to have a warming and nourishing effect on the *chi* energy. Traditional Chinese herbal remedies may also be prescribed (see the section on 'Herbal medicine') and simple dietary advice is commonly given.

Many parents are understandably nervous about using acupuncture for their children. They worry that the needles might frighten or hurt their child, or that there might be dangers if the child moves about. Practitioners say that, in practice, such problems rarely cause significant difficulties. However, if these matters concern you in particular, consider seeing a practitioner who specializes in work with children or who uses laser acupuncture (see below and page 50.

Western Acupuncture

Some doctors and physiotherapists practise what is called 'Western' acupuncture. This retains the mechanical components of acupuncture (needles, acupuncture points, etc.) but not its medical philosophy (*chi*, the five elements and so on). Western acupuncture might be offered by your GP or physiotherapist or in a conventional setting such as the pain clinic of a hospital. Its practice is somewhat different to that outlined above: for example, acupuncture points may be located using a special machine that measures the electrical resistance of the skin and diagnosis will take place along orthodox lines, rather than by using tongue and pulse diagnosis. See the section on 'Acupuncture in practice' (below) for more details.

Acupuncture Treatment

Some of the effects of acupuncture treatment are similar to those found in other complementary therapies. For example, most people feel well in themselves after a course of acupuncture treatment and they may find that they have more energy in daily life. Acupuncture has also been reported to be of benefit for recurrent infections, particularly colds and flu:

> Matthew had constant mucus congestion. He always had a cough, a runny nose, and infected eyes. After we started the acupuncture, we quickly noticed that the mucus dried up. His chest was clear and his coughing stopped. We also noticed that his breathing was less erratic and that he wasn't so prone to asthmatic wheezing.

This last point is particularly interesting: a number of scientific studies have indicated that acupuncture may be effective for asthma. In the treatment of cerebral palsy, however, most attention has centred on the possible role of acupuncture in relieving spasm and improving muscle tone and function. There is little doubt that, in some individuals at least, acupuncture can be of significant benefit. For example, the following cases were reported in a specialist medical journal.

1. During the last 3 years [an 18-year-old girl] has had recurrent episodes of pain in her back and flexion spasms of her left hip . . . acupuncture had a dramatic effect: the flexion spasm disappeared within 15 minutes. Altogether six such spasms have been treated, with the same drastic results, relapses being successively more infrequent.

2. A 12-year-old boy ... developed a rather painful flexion spasm of his left elbow. Almost complete remission was obtained after five treatments.
3. A 14-year-old boy ... had trouble with pain in his left shoulder and in the left side of his back. Muscle contractures and pain interfered with his walking ability. A few trials of acupuncture freed him completely of his trouble.
4. An 11-year-old girl with dystonic and hypertonic cerebral palsy ... developed peroneal muscle spasms, with corresponding foot deformities ... acupuncture treatment has led to successive improvement, with restoration of gait function [i.e. walking ability].

Dr Julian Kenyon, one of the British pioneers of laser acupuncture (see below), has worked with some 12 individuals with cerebral palsy. His primary goal has been to improve speech and he feels he has been successful in approximately half of his patients. One of his more dramatic cases involved a 3-year-old boy:

> After a couple of treatments, we began to notice a change in him. Previously, he was using speech patterns without being able to use words: just 'da da da'. But one day he came into the room where I was sitting and said 'I yuv you wummy.'

Many other practitioners have reported success at treating the physical problems of cerebral palsy, particularly when dealing with very young children. A number have also claimed positive effects for children with learning disability, be it associated with cerebral palsy, Down's syndrome, or other conditions:

> I worked with a number of learning disabled children when I was training in China. Acupuncture had the effect of "brightening up the mind": the children became more alert mentally.

There are a number of comments worth making about such claims. Firstly, they are essentially anecdotal in nature. So it is hard to know whether or not some of the changes noticed by acupuncturists and their patients would have happened in the absence of any treatment, or whether the benefits were really due to the acupuncture rather than any other therapy, for example, physiotherapy. There have been some trials of acupuncture for cerebral palsy, but though these have had favourable results, they did not conform to many of the basic standards of modern medical research. As a result, it is hard to draw any firm conclusions.

Secondly, improvements in learning disability are not widely reported by orthodox practitioners of acupuncture. This may be a function of the relationship non-medically qualified practitioners may build up with a family. Or it may be due to the fact that children who have problems with pain, spasm and recurrent flu are unlikely to be at their best for learning, and so any improvement in such problems may have knock-on effects on learning disability. Or it may be just wishful thinking.

There is some definite evidence, however, that acupuncture can have effects on epilepsy. Trials have been carried out in China, Sweden and the United States, and though these were not of high quality, a small pilot study in London is attempting to produce more evidence on the subject. There are some sound theoretical reasons for believing that acupuncture may be of benefit in epilepsy: one effect of needling is the release of a natural substance called GABA, which is similar to the chemicals used in anti-epileptic medication.

Acupuncture is based on the same principles as another complementary therapy, shiatsu (see also the section on page 96).

Acupuncture in Practice

The type of acupuncture described above is sometimes referred to as 'traditional acupuncture'. However, a number of orthodox physicians practise what is known as 'Western' acupuncture. Rather than assessing the energy state of meridians, the doctor makes an orthodox diagnosis and places needles in certain anatomical positions depending on the particular disease identified. The theory of Western acupuncture is rooted in standard anatomy and physiology: for example, researchers have linked acupuncture points to certain types of nerve endings and demonstrated that needling causes the release of natural pain-killing substances into the bloodstream.

Practitioners of traditional acupuncture say that because Western acupuncture foregoes the therapy's most basic theories and principles, it is not really acupuncture at all. Certainly the sort of acupuncture that GPs learn on a single weekend course might be considered to be a pale shadow of what can be achieved with this form of medicine.

On the other hand, using a conventional doctor does confer certain advantages. For example, doctor acupuncturists have a great grasp of basic medicine and can call on a battery of diagnostic laboratory tests: this might mean that they spot something requiring immediate action that a non-medically qualified acupuncturist might miss (however, you can avoid this problem by seeing both a practitioner of traditional acupuncture and your GP). Practitioners of Western acupuncture also point out that their practices are based on firm scientific research, rather than on tradition. Physiotherapists who practise acupuncture are able to integrate the technique within a wider rehabilitation programme. Finally, a relatively new form of acupuncture, laser acupuncture, is more widely practised by Western acupuncturists than by their traditional counterparts. In laser acupuncture, needles are replaced by a torch-like instrument that gives off a low-power laser beam when pressed against an acupuncture point. This method has several advantages: children are less frightened of the therapy, it is painless and it can be easier to use with people who have involuntary movements.

The section on 'Homoeopathy in practice' (page 124) has a full discussion of the pros and cons of conventionally trained and 'lay' practitioners of complementary medicine.

Acupuncture: a Summary

- Acupuncture is the insertion of fine needles through the skin for healing purposes.
- Acupuncture is said to be of benefit for recurrent infections such as colds and flu.
- There is increasing anecdotal evidence that acupuncture can improve muscle tone and function in cerebral palsy. This can be a long-term effect, particularly in young children. Speech has also been said to improve after acupuncture treatment.
- Acupuncture is widely regarded to be a valuable treatment for pain.
- Some practitioners also claim to be able to improve learning disability though there is some disagreement about this.
- Acupuncture is practised by doctors and physiotherapists, as well as by specialist practitioners.

Resources

Details of your local traditional acupuncturist are available from:

The Council for Acupuncture
179 Gloucester Place
London NW1 6DX
Tel: 071 724 5756

This register also lists practitioners who also use Chinese Herbalism (see the section on 'Herbal medicine', page 127). If you are particularly interested in one or other of these forms of traditional Chinese medicine, you should state this when you contact the council.

Details of practitioners who have experience of work with children are kept by the:

Children's Acupuncture Register
City Health Centre
36–37 Featherstone Street
London EC1Y 8QX

If you do decide that you want to see a doctor, contact:

The British Medical Acupuncture Society
Newton House, Newton Lane
Lower Whitley, Warrington
Cheshire
Tel: 0925 730727

A large number of physiotherapists now practise acupuncture. Details are kept by the:

Acupuncture Association of Chartered Physiotherapists
Bow House Physiotherapy Practice
Bow Street
Lang Port
Somerset TA10 9PQ.

SHIATSU

Introduction to Shiatsu

Shiatsu is the one of the more widely established therapies that uses *acupressure*, the manipulation of acupuncture points with the fingers. Though there are a number of different forms of acupressure, few, if any, have developed the coherence of method and philosophy that is found in shiatsu.

Shiatsu developed earlier in this century in Japan, and its basic concepts borrow heavily from traditional Oriental medicine (see the section on 'Acupuncture'). Health is seen to depend on the correct flow of *chi* energy through the body; ideas such as the meridians, the five elements and the pulses are also retained. However, there are several important differences between acupuncture and shiatsu. Firstly, because fingers replace needles as the primary means of affecting the flow of *chi*, the experience of shiatsu is much more personal than that of acupuncture, with the practitioner more intimately involved in treatment. Another difference is that whereas an acupuncturist will needle perhaps two or three locations during a session, a shiatsu practitioner will generally cover the whole body, though a few particular areas may be given special attention. Finally, an acupuncturist will generally attempt to make a precise diagnosis; a shiatsu practitioner is more likely to assess the 'feel' of a client and go along with that.

In general, just as acupuncture tends towards the more rational and exact, shiatsu tends towards the more intuitive and personal. In many ways, shiatsu may be regarded as a half-way house between massage and acupuncture: the use of touch, the involvement of the whole body and the more instinctive approach to diagnosis and treatment are important elements of massage; the concepts of meridians and *chi* and the use of special points on the body to bring about specific changes are principles found in acupuncture.

Visiting a Practitioner

Unlike most complementary therapies, in which special treatment couches are used, shiatsu practitioners work with their clients on a thick mat on the floor. They also work through clothes: clients should wear something light and preferably baggy to a shiatsu session. After a brief chat and case history, the client removes shoes and any heavy outer clothing and lies or sits on the floor. The practitioner starts work fairly quickly: in shiatsu, diagnosis takes place during treatment.

If applied carefully, finger pressure on the *tsubo* (the shiatsu name for acupuncture points) should not be painful. There is a feeling of heaviness and often one of well-being. Though these sensations are distinct, and though the practitioner may move your limbs and body during treatment, shiatsu treatment is generally very relaxing.

Shiatsu Treatment

Shiatsu combines elements of both massage and acupuncture, so it is not surprising that the effects of shiatsu treatment include benefits associated with both of these therapies. In common with massage, shiatsu can ease muscular stiffness and tension, improve blood circulation and bring many of the benefits of human touch. In common with acupuncture, shiatsu is able to promote more specific changes in the body.

A particularly interesting shiatsu case history is that of Anton, who has cerebral palsy and is a wheelchair user. Anton has written this of his 18 months' experience with shiatsu:

> At the start of this year I was in so much pain in my body. I was uncomfortable sitting in my wheelchair, I was sitting badly leaning over on one side. I felt generally unwell and I was losing all the confidence I had. I felt quite unhappy.
>
> Since I have been having shiatsu, I feel so different in my body. I don't often get tense in my limbs and if I do, I know it will go away. I don't get pain in my left leg when I am using my computer now. I feel more solid in my wheelchair. I rarely get that terrible pain in my stomach.
>
> I am eating very well, I feel stronger, I am sleeping good. I am happier, I still get my off-days but as my parents said, most people get their off-days. I am relaxed and I feel great.

Anton's practitioner also noticed that though he normally had four or five colds during winter, he had only one in the entire period of his treatment. Anton noted that he now recovers more rapidly from the infections he does get.

For reasons that are not entirely clear, shiatsu practitioners in the UK have not tended to work with children. This may be seen as unusual, especially as acupressure therapy is apparently widely used for disabled children in mainland China. A Chinese doctor who specializes in rehabilitation, Professor Wang Zhao-Pu, has recently published a book about acupressure for neurological disabilities (see Further Reading). In the book he gives a number of case histories of children with cerebral palsy. Though as many as seventy or eighty treatment sessions were often required, the results of therapy appeared to be good, especially with moderately disabled children:

> The patient walked with a limp and a slight sluggish gait, the right foot dropped and moved in a circular motion, and the right elbow was flexed and had a fixed posture during gross motor activities . . . [after treatment] he walked and ran without a limp or sluggish gait. He moved his right arm while walking. He had reasonable voluntary control over his right arm and hand . . .

It is important to note that Zhao-Pu uses acupressure as part of a wider approach, one which includes physiotherapy manipulations, exercises and the use of splints. Certainly the average shiatsu practitioner is unlikely to have the experience, the training and the special expertise in disability of Zhao-Pu. However, as the case of Anton shows, such practitioners can often offer a valuable service and it will be interesting to see how the practice of shiatsu with children develops over the course of the next few years.

Shiatsu in Practice

The Shiatsu Society has an excellently controlled register, though not all competent practitioners are listed.

Shiatsu needs no special equipment and it is thus especially easy for practitioners to do outcalls.

Shiatsu: a Summary

- Shiatsu is based on similar principles to acupuncture except that it is fingers rather than needles that are used on the acupuncture points.
- Shiatsu shares a number of benefits with massage including improving blood circulation and easing stiffness and tension in the short term. There are also the benefits of human touch.
- Shiatsu may also be able to bring about more specific changes in function and muscle tone.

Resources

The Shiatsu Society
5 Foxcote
Wokingham
Berkshire RG11 3PG
Tel: 0734 730836

STRUCTURAL TECHNIQUES

OSTEOPATHY AND CHIROPRACTIC

Many people are aware that osteopathy and chiropractic are similar therapies, in fact, the founder of chiropractic, Daniel D. Palmer, originally trained with the founder of osteopathy, Andrew Taylor Still. In modern times, the two professions remain so comparable that a significant proportion of textbooks and journals are relevant to both. As the effects of osteopathic and chiropractic treatment are similar, they will be considered together. As there are more osteopaths than chiropractors in the UK, and because it is more common to find osteopaths working with children, only osteopathy will be discussed below. However, this section should also be seen as referring to chiropractic.

Introduction to Osteopathy

Osteopathy is a therapy of the physical structures of the body. Whereas acupuncturists and healers work with energy, and whereas herbalists and homoeopaths work (presumably) at a chemical level, osteopaths work with bones, muscles and connective tissue, using their hands to diagnose and treat abnormalities of structure and function.

Osteopathy is perhaps best explained by looking at one of its most well-known applications: the treatment of back pain. An osteopath examining a person with back pain will look for vertebra (the bones of the spine) that have unusual ranges of motion. These are thought to cause pain by impinging on nerves, something that can result in muscle spasm. Typically, an osteopath will use what is known as a 'high velocity thrust', or 'manipulation', to correct such a problem. Popularly known as 'cracking a joint', this technique involves a short, sharp motion designed to free up structures that are adhering to one another. Osteopaths believe that once the bones of the spine are correctly aligned, the body's own healing and recuperative mechanisms will come in to play and lead to relief from back pain.

Manipulation is only one of a number of techniques that osteopaths use to improve the structure and mechanics of the body. Other common osteopathic procedures include mobilization, a form of stretching, and soft-tissue work, which is somewhat similar to massage.

In work with children, however, such techniques generally form only a minor part of osteopathic therapy. What is more common is the use of what are known as functional techniques. Functional techniques can best be described using the example of a stiff shoulder. In manipulation or mobilization the osteopath would use a forceful man-oeuvre to improve the mobility of the joint; in functional work, the arm might be gently moved within the shoulder joint's range of motion. Osteopaths say that, in functional techniques, the body responds to the practitioner's touch in such a way as to rectify abnormalities of its own accord.

Probably the most important and high profile functional technique is cranial osteopathy, or cranio-sacral therapy as it is sometimes known. Cranial osteopathy focuses on the nervous system. Practitioners place their hands on the skull bones (the cranium) and the flat bone at the base of the spine (the sacrum) of the client and feel for a rhythm that they say it is possible to detect. By working with this rhythm, and by gently handling the bones of the skull, osteopaths say that they can balance disturbances and distortions in the nervous system.

Cranial osteopathy has become such a popular technique that some practitioners use it almost exclusively. In fact, in the minds of many, cranial osteopathy is synonymous with the osteopathic treatment of children. See the section on 'Osteopathy and chiropractic in practice' (page 106) for more details.

Visiting an Osteopath

Exactly what happens during a session of osteopathy depends on whether the practitioner is intending to use manipulation, or whether only cranial techniques will be used. In the former case, the client undresses to his or her underwear so that the practitioner can observe the structure of the bones and muscles. The practitioner makes further examinations by use of the hands and assesses the mobility of various parts of the body by asking the client to

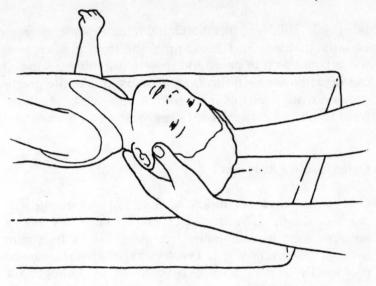

Figure 3. A child receiving cranial osteopathy.

make a few simple movements, for example, bending to one side or twisting.

Treatment takes place on a low couch. Most of a session may be taken up with work on the soft tissues (the skin, muscles and connective tissue) to prepare for the manipulation. The practitioner places the client in position using pillows and makes a short and precise thrust to complete the manoeuvre.

In cranial osteopathy, there is less need for the practitioner to make a precise visual examination of the mobility and structure of the body. After the case history, the client lays on the treatment couch (there is no need to undress) and the practitioner starts work right away. The treatment is very gentle and subtle: in fact, it is not immediately apparent to someone watching a session that any form of therapy is taking place. For the client, cranial osteopathy is a very gentle and soothing experience: some people say that they feel energy moving around, a little like healing.

Some people also experience some form of emotional

release. In children, this emotional release can sometimes be quite distressing. For example, the child may cry and move about as if in panic and may refuse to be treated. It can occasionally be difficult for parents to take the practitioner's word that this is a positive sign. Such situations need to be approached with some care.

Osteopathic Treatment

Osteopathy involves touch so it is not surprising that many of the benefits found in therapies such as massage are also seen in osteopathy (see page 64). A treatment session, particularly if it involves cranial work, can be profoundly relaxing and pleasurable. Many parents have noticed that their children remain unusually still and quiet during cranial osteopathy. Touch can also lead to greater body awareness and improved self-esteem (see page 63).

Osteopaths say that their extended training gives them an advantage over massage practitioners when it comes to the careful and directed use of touch, particularly with disabled people:

> Osteopaths are professionals at touching and they use touch in a very special way. This touch can be very subtle and penetrating.

Osteopaths also say that their training gives them an advantage in maximizing some of the other benefits of touch discussed in the section on massage. These include short-term effects on pain, spasm, physical mobility, behaviour and symptoms of the digestive tract such as indigestion and constipation.

However, for many people, especially those parents who visit institutions such as the Osteopathic Centre for Children (see below), what is of prime interest is whether osteopathy can bring about long-term changes in the physical and mental functioning of children.

This question is dealt with at some length in Chapter 2

(page 26). To recap: though there are numerous problems in trying to assess the effects of complementary therapy in disabled children, and though there has not been sufficient scientific research to decide the matter, there is accumulating anecdotal evidence that suggests that osteopathy can be of long-term benefit in at least some children.

Brian is a GP based in London. His son Tim was diagnosed as having cerebral palsy at the age of 4 months when a scan revealed intracerebral bleeding and hydrocephalus. Tim was taken to an osteopath regularly for over a year and his doctors have been pleased with his progress:

> The neurologist says that Tim is doing better than expected. He certainly is doing very well: the work seems to have helped with his squint and with his mobility and muscle function. When he was assessed at 20 months, he was found to have normal cognitive and social functioning and gross motor skills at the very lower limit of the normal range.

Brian points out that because Tim was also receiving conventional physiotherapy, homoeopathy and conductive education, it is difficult to tell for sure whether the osteopathy itself was of benefit. Other parents, however, appear not to have this problem:

> During the third treatment session, the practitioner said that she had finally been able to make some real changes. A few days after that, Danny started to walk on his own. It was all of a sudden and it took the physio completely by surprise. Seeing as how we'd continued on other therapies as normal, it is hard to believe that it wasn't the osteopathy that caused the improvement.

For some children, the benefit seems to be primarily mental and behavioural, rather than physical:

> Two months after the onset of treatment, Robert had a routine appointment with the paediatrician who commented to his mother that he could not believe the difference in Robert's behaviour during the consultation.

Robert also experienced a significant decrease in the frequency and severity of seizures after treatment and this led the paediatrician to reduce the level of anti-convulsant medication.

Some workers have claimed that osteopathy may be particularly indicated in Down's syndrome. This condition is marked by changes to the structure of the skull. At least some of these changes, for example, the flattening of the nasal sinuses, are known to lead to health difficulties. It is quite possible that a therapy such as cranial osteopathy, which focuses on correcting the structural abnormalities of the skull, may be of benefit. Some osteopaths have reported good results and the use of cranial osteopathy in Down's syndrome appears to be increasing: in New Zealand it is common for osteopaths to work alongside orthodox health professionals in what is called an 'Early Intervention Team'.

The reputed benefits of osteopathy for cerebral palsy and other disabilities clearly call for some rigorous research to be conducted. Though some initial preliminary work has been completed (see page 28) it is clear that only a large, well-conducted trial will be able to decide whether osteopathy is of long-term benefit for disabled children.

Osteopathy and Chiropractic in Practice

As pointed out in the introduction to this section, osteopathy and chiropractic are distinct, if similar, therapies. The differences between the two techniques are subtle. For example, whereas chiropractors pay detailed attention to the local mechanics of the spine, osteopaths are more inclined to look at a person's overall posture and mobility. It can be difficult for clients to tell how such differences will affect them and, as ever, making a decision will be a case of choosing the right practitioner, rather than the right therapy.

However, there are various issues that become important when disability is involved. Firstly, because osteopathic and chiropractic work with disabled children is predominantly a matter of cranial therapy, it is worth checking how much cranial work, if any, a potential practitioner uses. It certainly appears to be more common among osteopaths than chiropractors.

It is also worth knowing that there are two different types of chiropractic in the UK: McTimoney and regular. McTimoney chiropractors say that their method is more gentle and less invasive than standard practice: they also say that they always look at the whole body, rather than concentrating on specific sections of the spine. Regular chiropractors say that their standards of training and qualification are higher than in McTimoney chiropractic and that it is more effective to work on specific areas of the body than to try to cover the entire skeleton.

Osteopathy and Chiropractic: a Summary

- Osteopathy and chiropractic are therapies of the musculo-skeletal system of the body.
- Though osteopaths and chiropractors are most well-known for 'cracking backs', their work with disabled children is predominantly a matter of cranial therapy, a rather more gentle technique.
- Osteopathy and chiropractic can be used to bring about physical benefits such as short-term effects on blood circulation, constipation and pain.
- Osteopathy and chiropractic are also said to be able to bring about long-term improvements in physical and mental functioning in some disabled children. However, it is not known for sure whether the therapies do indeed have this effect.

Resources

The General Council and Register of Osteopaths
56 London Street
Reading
Berks RG1 4SQ
Tel: 0734 576585/566260

The GCRO has ensured that osteopathy is probably the most well-regulated of the complementary therapies. It runs an excellent referral service.

Osteopathic Centre for Children (OCC)
4 Harcourt House
19a Cavendish Square
London W1M 9AD
Tel: 071 495 1231

The OCC provides osteopathic services for children in a clinic format. Appointment fees are low and there is a sliding scale of fees.

For a McTimoney practitioner, SAE to:

The Institute of Pure Chiropractic
14 Park End Street
Oxford OX1 1HH
Tel: 0865 246687

For a regular chiropractor, SAE to:

British Chiropractic Association
29 Whitley Street
Reading RG2 0EG
Tel: 0734 757557

If you include £1 in your SAE, you will be sent a full register plus a variety of leaflets and other information.

Your GP might also be able to refer you to an appropriate local osteopath or chiropractor.

Legislation is being prepared to pave the way for statutory regulation of the manipulative therapies, which is due to come in to effect in 1996. It is likely that this will inprove standards of practice and consumer choice: however, some of these comments on practice and resources may become out of date.

ROLFING

Rolfing is named after its originator, Ida Rolf, though she herself preferred the title 'Structural Integration'. The aim of the technique is to align the body in an optimal position with respect to gravity, something which allows a person to stand erect, and make other movements, with less muscular effort.

The work itself consists of a cycle of ten one-hour sessions, each focusing on a different area of the body. Strong pressure is applied with the hands to parts of the body where muscle tendons are felt to adhere to each other, rather than slide over one another in a normal way. As such, Rolfing is comparable to osteopathy and chiropractic, except whereas practitioners of the latter manipulate bones, Rolfers manipulate soft tissue. Another difference is that whereas osteopaths and chiropractors will seek to locate and remedy specific faults, Rolfers always work on the whole body: the ten-session cycle is used regardless of the client's state of well-being.

The pressure used in Rolfing is firm enough to cause pain, but this is often accompanied by a sense of well-being and emotional release. This is explained as follows: when we experience emotions such as anxiety, depression or fear we tense our muscles in characteristic ways. Sometimes, patterns of muscle-use associated with emotions become habitual, almost as if the emotion has become 'locked in' to the body. Rolfers say that their work can help release these locked in emotions and a number have reported on psychological changes in children with disabilities such as autism.

Rolfers believe that they can help conditions such as cerebral palsy because the therapy can help improve flexibility and mobility, typically leaving clients feeling 'freer and lighter'. Some evidence supporting these claims comes from a scientific study conducted in the United States in 1981. The researchers found that the effectiveness of Rolfing depended on the severity of the disability: for children with severe disability, no improvements were observed; those who were 'moderately' affected experienced some improvements in flexibility and strength, though not enough to make a significant impact on their ability to walk. However, for younger, mildly affected children, Rolfing did appear to lead to measurable improvements in walking ability.

Rolfing is a relatively new therapy. It is more predominant in the United States, where it is popular among physiotherapists. There are only a dozen or so practitioners in the UK, primarily in London and the south-east.

Resources

Rolf Institute
PO BOX 1868
Boulder CO 80306-1868
USA
Tel: 303 449 5903

The British contact for Rolfers is Jenny Crewdson who can be reached on 071 834 1493.

FUNCTIONAL TECHNIQUES

THE ALEXANDER TECHNIQUE

The Alexander technique teaches individuals to use themselves more effectively in everyday life. Practitioners of the technique say that every movement we make and every posture we adopt constitutes a 'use' of the body. The purpose of the Alexander technique is to teach 'good use', the principle of which is that movement should involve a lengthening and widening of the body and the absence of unnecessary muscle tension, especially in the neck. Teachers of the Alexander technique are particularly interested in helping their pupils identify the habits that interfere with the body's natural functioning and co-ordination. Helping a person to recognize and 'inhibit' these habits is seen as one of the main purposes of an Alexander session.

The Alexander technique is taught by using simple activities as a starting point. For example, a lesson may focus on lying down or getting out of a chair. Teachers give verbal directions, such as 'allow your head to ease gently up from your spine', and use their hands to guide the pupil and bring their attention to particular parts of the body. In this way the pupil comes to recognize the habitual patterns whereby they have been misusing their body and, as an Alexander teacher might put it, be given the choice of a better use.

For Adigwe, a 35-year-old with mild cerebral palsy, this was one of the main benefits of the Alexander technique:

> I've found it quite useful as a coaching and correcting process for overcoming bad habits. My centre of gravity tends to come forward, and I'm often walking on tip-toe with my left leg twisting in. The Alexander technique has made me more conscious of my centre of gravity.

Adigwe also raised the point that, as an Alexander teacher might put it: 'Use affects functioning.' To give a simple example, it is easier to lift a heavy book off a desk by moving close to it and using both arms than by stretching out and using one arm as a long lever:

> I was consuming a lot of energy just to walk. I am now more even.

Others have found that Alexander lessons have led to relief from pain. Karen, an adult with mild cerebral palsy, came to an Alexander teacher complaining of pain in her legs. She took regular lessons over the course of a year. Her teacher says that by learning better use of her body, Karen overcame the habits that caused the tightening and twisting of her leg muscles that gave her pain. Karen herself is less positive that the Alexander technique led to relief from the leg pains – after all, who is to know whether they would have got better anyway? – but she continues to visit her Alexander teacher:

> It has made me aware of my body, how I am sitting or standing. It's a very slow and subtle change. But I do find that I am calmer, and that I don't jump so much at unexpected noises.

In many ways, Alexander technique is a method of learning, as opposed to a therapy. The benefits of the technique are felt once a pupil incorporates its principles into everyday life. Learning how to sit, stand and move more efficiently will only bring improved performance, and relief from pain, if what is learned is used outside the context of the lesson. Though this emphasis on self-help is to be applauded, difficulties do arise in the use of the technique with young children and those with learning or communication difficulties. In disability work, the predominant group using the Alexander technique are adults with physical disabilities, particularly where these are relatively mild.

More detailed information on the Alexander technique can be found in *Complementary Medicine and Disability* (see Further Reading).

Resources

Society of Teachers of the Alexander Technique
20 London House
266 Fulham Road
London SW10 9EL
Tel: 071 351 0828

FELDENKRAIS

Feldenkrais is a technique whereby individuals can be taught to become more aware of their bodies and hence move and function more efficiently. As such, there are many parallels between Feldenkrais and the Alexander technique. Both methods work not with the structure of the body, as an osteopath would, but with its function. Alexander teachers talk about 'use' of the body; Feldenkrais workers focus on movement.

Feldenkrais work incorporates two separate elements: Awareness Through Movement and Functional Integration. Awareness Through Movement takes the form of a class practising special sets of small and unusual movements. For example, while sitting in a chair, a person might move one knee at a time gently forward while turning the head to one side, sometimes the same side as the knee, other times the opposite side.

Functional Integration is the hands-on part of Feldenkrais. The client lies passively on a low couch and the practitioner uses small, slow and gentle movements of the client's body. For example, a hard flat surface such as a book may be lightly pressed against the sole of the foot and tilted in various directions. With young children, and for others who may find 'Awareness Through Movement' difficult, 'Functional Integration' will be the predominant means of treatment.

Feldenkrais practitioners believe that the body has an inherent ability to organize itself into movement. The aim of Awareness Through Movement and Functional Integration is to facilitate this process. Practitioners say that if the nervous system is allowed to experience various different forms of movement in subtle variations it will recognize for itself the most appropriate and efficient way of moving.

It is clear that Feldenkrais is very different from therapies such as Doman-Delcato (see page 151) that attempt to impose a developmental pattern and inhibit 'unhealthy' reflexes. For example, Moshe Feldenkrais, the originator of the technique, once worked with a child with cerebral palsy whose legs had contracted together so that they touched. Instead of trying to force the limbs apart, Feldenkrais gently pressed them even closer, almost as if he was telling the nervous system: 'Look, this is how the body is!' and allowing it to release the spasticity for itself.

Moshe Feldenkrais was particularly interested in the problems of adults and children with damage to the nervous system and this interest has remained among modern practitioners. For example, a recent issue of the Feldenkrais Journal UK was dedicated exclusively to this topic. One article relates the personal story of Paul Doron-Doroftei, who first experienced Feldenkrais as an adolescent with cerebral palsy and later became a teacher of the technique. He now works in Germany and concentrates on the treatment of disabled children.

There is little doubt that Feldenkrais might have much to offer to people with disabilities such as cerebral palsy. However, the work does have a drawback: its youth. The first training for practitioners took place in the mid-1970s and the first British programme did not see its first graduates until 1990. So it is likely that appropriate standards of training and qualification are yet to be firmly established and that most practitioners will have relatively little experience of practise, particularly with people who are disabled. Furthermore, at the current time of writing, Feldenkrais has yet to be evaluated by scientific trial.

Resources

Feldenkrais Guild
PO BOX 370
London N10 3XA

SELF-HELP DISCIPLINES

'Complementary medicine' and 'complementary therapies' are often used as interchangeable terms. However, at least some of the techniques in complementary medicine aren't really therapies, something done to you by a practitioner, but disciplines, something you learn and practice for yourself. Many people see the self-help nature of techniques such as yoga and meditation as liberating and empowering:

> It is a way of doing something positive for myself, and I don't have to depend on other people or props of any kind.

However, self-help techniques can sometimes be difficult to use with young children or with people who have learning or communication difficulties. Some applications do seem to be successful: for example, yoga and relaxation techniques are used widely with adults who have learning disabilities. Other practices, such as tai chi for children, do not appear to have gained in popularity.

MEDITATION AND RELAXATION TECHNIQUES

Various methods have been developed to calm the body and still the mind. Many meditation techniques stem from the spiritual practices of the East; other relaxation exercises were designed by Western doctors as a specific cure for stress-related illness.

In general, meditation focuses on the mind: the meditation may involve focusing attention on the breath or on a 'mantra', a special word that is repeated over and over. Great importance is placed on allowing the mind to become empty of thought.

Relaxation techniques tend to focus on the body. One widely used relaxation technique is known as 'progressive muscle relaxation' in which sets of muscles are held taut for 15 seconds or so and then allowed to relax. In theory, mental quietness and relaxation stem from this physical relaxation.

Meditation and relaxation techniques have been found to reduce spasm and spasticity. In one study, a group of adults with cerebral palsy were able to complete a manual task more effectively after a course of relaxation. Other trials have shown that relaxation techniques reduce disruptive behaviours in adults with learning disabilities. This result would probably not surprise those individuals who have found that problems of muscle tone (and disruptive behaviour) are exacerbated by stress and anxiety.

Other individuals have found that the effects of taking up meditation and relaxation techniques have been more subtle. Ruth, a 30-year-old woman who has cerebral palsy, has said this of her experiences:

> Meditation put me in touch with myself. And I discovered that I was not my physical body, that I was not equal to, and bound by, this thing that other people called "deformed". Meditation became a relaxing and refreshing break.

But it would be a mistake to see the effects of meditation and relaxation purely in terms of the 'special problems' of disabled people. Most people take up meditation for reasons entirely unconnected with specific health difficulties. For instance, meditation feels good: it is deeply relaxing and enjoyable. Some people say that they love the way that meditation allows them to 'sign out' from all the hassles and petty aggravations and take time to be with themselves. Others say that meditation calms them and helps clear their mind. Most people who meditate consistently will say that the calmness and self-awareness experienced during meditation spill out into their entire lives.

In short, relaxation and meditation techniques can promote physical and psychological well-being regardless of an individual's level ability or disability. It is of interest, for example, that the comment below might just as well have come from the husband of a harassed business-woman as from the mother of a disabled child:

> The change in her has been enormous, and the rest of the family know immediately if she has forgotten to meditate. Even friends who did not know she was meditating have mentioned how much calmer Lucinda is now.

YOGA AND TAI CHI

Yoga and tai chi combine movement and postures with breathing and meditation work. As such, yoga and tai chi have been seen to be especially appropriate for people who have physical disabilities. It is widely recognized that exercise is important for health: yoga and tai chi combine exercise with a number of features that some disabled people have found particularly attractive. Perhaps most importantly, yoga and tai chi feel good. Many people say that they enjoy the graceful and flowing movements of yoga and tai chi and that they feel peaceful and relaxed, rather than worn out, at the end of the session.

An issue of particular importance seems to be that of body awareness. Many of the exercises in yoga and tai chi are concerned with improving an individual's awareness of their body. The slow movements in tai chi, for example, require a person to have a greater understanding of his or her body than might be required by the rapid, habitual movements of everyday life. In yoga, great attention is placed on the breath and the energy within the body:

> Yoga heightens my awareness of my body in a conscious way.

> I wish my parents had sent me when I was young. You learn about your balance and posture. It gives you an inner confidence.

Complementary Medicine and Disability (see Further Reading) contains more detailed information about yoga, tai chi and meditation/relaxation.

Yoga, Tai Chi and Meditation in Practice

Yoga, tai chi and meditation/relaxation are generally taught to groups. Many adult education authorities run classes on weekday evenings during term time; other classes are available at natural health centres or are advertised in local newspapers or magazines. Though such classes might well be appropriate for adults and older children with milder disabilities, other individuals, such as children or those with severe disabilities, might well require more specialist teaching.

Local social services often run yoga or relaxation classes aimed at specific client groups. Alternatively, the organizations listed below can be a useful resource in finding specialist teachers.

Resources

Send SAEs to:

Yoga
The Yoga for Health Foundation
Ickwell Bury, Biggleswade
Bedfordshire SG18 9EF
Tel: 076 727 271
Residential yoga courses. Many disabled people visit Ickwell Bury. The foundation also publishes a list of teachers throughout the country.

You and Me Yoga Centre
The Cottage, Burton in Kendal
Carnforth
Lancs LA6 1ND
Yoga and special needs.

The British Wheel of Yoga
1 Hamilton Place
Boston Road
Sleaford
Lincs NG34 7ES
Tel: 0529 306851

Iyengar Yoga Institute
223a Randolph Avenue
London W9 1NL
Tel: 071 624 3080

Yoga Biomedical Trust
PO Box 140
Cambridge CB1 1PU
Can provide contact addresses for yoga therapists
throughout the country for a £3 charge. Yoga therapists
use exercises that are designed to aid the treatment of
specific conditions.

Tai Chi
Village Hall Tai Chi
163 Palatine Road
Manchester M20 8GH
A centre of information and advice about tai chi for people
who have special needs.

British Tai Chi Chuan Association
7 Upper Wimpole Street
London W1
Tel: 071 935 8444

Tai Chi Union for Great Britain
Ray Wilkie
Secretary
23 Oakwood Avenue
Mitcham
Surrey CR4 3DQ

Tai Chi North
Chris Thomas
Secretary
131 Tunstall Road
Knypersley
Stoke-on-Trent ST8 7AA
Tai chi instructors in the north of England and Scotland.

Meditation/relaxation:
Relaxation for Living
Dunesk
Burwood Park Road
Walton on Thames
Surrey KY12 5LH

Autogenic Training
101 Harley Street
London W1N 1DF

ORALLY TAKEN REMEDIES

HOMOEOPATHY

Introduction to Homoeopathy

Homoeopaths treat illness by using extremely small doses of common substances in pill form. In this respect, homoeopathy is somewhat like visiting an orthodox physician: the practitioner takes a case history and gives you some medicine to take.

Homoeopathy was founded in the late eighteenth century by Dr Samuel Hahnemann. Hahnemann discovered that quinine, the cure for malaria, causes the symptoms of malaria in a healthy person. By a series of experiments, in which he prepared remedies from dilute solutions of natural materials, he formulated the principle of 'let like be cured with like': small doses of a substance remedy the symptoms that are caused by a large dose of that substance.

Modern homoeopathy is still very much governed by Hahnemann's basic principles. Homoeopaths believe that human beings have an inherent ability to heal themselves and that homoeopathic remedies stimulate this process. This is why remedies are prescribed depending on the particular characteristics of each individual, rather than the disease: it is common for two people with precisely the same medical condition to be given different homoeopathic preparations.

Homoeopathic medicine is generally free from unwanted side-effects and though some say that it is hard to see why it should work, there is much scientific evidence in its favour (see page 9 in Chapter 1). Homoeopathy is recognized by the NHS and there are a number of hospitals that specialize in homoeopathic medicine. On the continent, homoeopathy is even more popular: in France and Germany, there are more than 10,000 orthodox doctors using homoeopathy.

Visiting a Homoeopath

The first visit to a homoeopath is generally the longest, with the initial case history taking between an hour and an hour and a half. The homoeopath needs to know the exact details of an individual's symptoms, for example, how they are affected by the weather. Other questions can include an individual's sleeping patterns, emotional reactions or even taste in food. All in all, the homoeopath will try to make an assessment of the client's entire mental, physical and emotional state. This 'constitutional type' is the basis for choosing the most appropriate remedy.

Taking a child's homoeopathic case history can be a little bit more difficult as children may not be able to answer direct questions about, for example, their emotions. The homoeopath will try to build up a picture by questioning the parent, and, if possible, by asking the child indirect questions about toys, hobbies or television programmes. Observing the child at rest and play can also provide an experienced homoeopath with useful information.

After writing the prescription, the homoeopath will give advice on taking the medication, for example, it is necessary to avoid coffee and camphor, and arrange for a second appointment. A course of homoeopathic treatment involves several appointments, particularly in chronic or serious conditions. The homoeopath will assess your or your child's progress at each appointment and, if needed, prescribe new remedies or 'potencies' (different potencies reflect different dilutions of a remedy). It may take several attempts for the homoeopath to find the right remedy, on the other hand, you might get lucky straightaway and in this case, a further visit to the homoeopath might bring no change in treatment. Some people feel slightly cheated if this happens as they may have had to pay good money just to be nodded at and told to wait and see. However, that is just a fact of homoeopathic treatment.

One thing to watch out for is an 'aggravation reaction' when symptoms worsen for a few days. This is a sign that the homoeopathic medicine is working and is generally harmless. However, in certain conditions, for example, asthma or epilepsy, aggravations can potentially cause some difficulties and this is something worth discussing with your homoeopath.

Modern homoeopaths prescribe in various ways. In 'classical homoeopathy', the aim of treatment is to find the one single remedy most appropriate for the individual, but some homoeopaths vary this by prescribing more than one remedy or by practising 'polypharmacy', where several homoeopathic medicines are combined in a single pill. One non-classical practice that can be very useful for disabled people is the prescribing of remedies to be used 'as required' for recurring symptoms. This is something worth discussing with your homoeopath: obviously they will try to help you or your child improve to the point where symptoms no longer do recur, but this may not be possible. In this case, your homoeopath could prescribe remedies to be kept for use whenever a certain symptom flares up (an 'acute standby'). Being able to resort to a harmless and non-addictive treatment for recurring symptoms is something that many people find a particularly attractive feature of homoeopathy.

Homoeopathic Treatment

The primary use of homeopathy in the treatment of people who have cerebral palsy or similar conditions is in the control of recurrent secondary symptoms:

> Philip used to be clogged up and flu-ey constantly in the winter. He's only had about one or two minor colds since we started the homoeopathy.

> She started getting the ear infections when she was about two-and-a-half, after which she was on antibiotics for two years. Homoeopathic treatment has helped tremendously. The infections are much rarer now and when they do come back, we can clear them up almost immediately with homoeopathy.

A common experience is that treatment falls into three stages. Firstly, there may be very little effect at all as a number of different remedies are tried. Eventually, an appropriate remedy is found and, after a course of treatment, the frequency of attacks of the symptom decreases, sometimes dramatically. Finally, homoeopathy is used to treat the symptom when it does recur, often bringing relatively rapid relief.

Symptoms that are common in disabled adults and children and that homoeopaths are confident of treating include: sleep difficulties, urinary tract infections, constipation, diarrhoea, colic, vomiting, respiratory infections (flu and colds), ear infections, 'glue ear', poor circulation and muscle pain.

Some homoeopaths also claim to have been able to treat the primary symptoms in certain classes of disability. One of the areas that has received most attention is learning disability: there are a number of reports where improvements in alertness, concentration, behaviour and ability have followed homoeopathic therapy. For example, the parents of a child with Down's syndrome have made the following comments:

> The homoeopathy has brought her into the world. She is somehow more present, bright and focused. When the pills run out, she gradually withdraws again.

There have also been reports of benefit in epilepsy, although homoeopathic treatment, and the assessment of its outcome, is often complicated by the effects of anti-epileptic medication. Somewhat less is known about the use of homoeopathy to treat problems of movement and muscle tone. Some homoeopaths say that there are remedies for 'stiffness' (that is, spasticity) and that hypotonia (flaccid muscles), involuntary movements such as athetosis, and ataxia (incoordination) can sometimes be moderated to a degree.

However, others are less sure that changes in learning or muscle tone can be brought about by homoeopathy, in fact, the whole area is somewhat controversial. Certainly what is more commonly noted is the relief of secondary symptoms (such as recurrent flu) and perhaps above all, an increase in general well-being:

> Sam is generally stronger and healthier nowadays. He used to be so sickly before we went to see the homoeopath.

> I feel so much better in myself: my constipation is completely gone and my appetite is much improved. ... I have more energy.

Homoeopathy in Practice

There are two categories of homoeopaths: homoeopathic physicians, or 'doctor homoeopaths', who learn homoeopathy having completed an orthodox medical education, and 'lay homoeopaths', who practise without formal medical qualifications. Each has its own particular advantages.

Doctor homoeopaths obviously have a greater grasp of basic medicine and there are certain times when this is particularly relevant. For example, homoeopathy often causes an aggravation of symptoms in the early stages of treatment, and in some conditions, for example, asthma or epilepsy, such an aggravation can have serious consequences. A homoeopathic physician might also be indicated if you or your child are taking drugs of any kind, particularly if you are interested in reducing the dosage as a result of homoeopathic treatment: sometimes drugs are used to suppress a condition (for example, epilepsy) in such a way that it can be difficult to tell how the condition is being affected by treatment; moreover, it can sometimes be difficult to prescribe homoeopathically for people who are taking drugs. Finally, if you are not sure about you or your child's symptoms, a medically qualified homoeopath can be of enormous help, especially as he or she may have access to laboratory tests, X-rays and so on. Some symptoms are not what they seem and a doctor homoeopath is in a good position to spot whether a particular symptom needs checking out.

One of the main reasons people give for preferring lay homoeopaths is that they feel they can have a more natural relationship than with a homoeopathic GP. Doctor homoeopaths are sometimes seen to be much like any other doctors in terms of their relationship with their clients. For example, they often use terms such as 'spastics' or 'Down's patients'; lay homoeopaths are much more likely to talk of particular people who have particular problems. Perhaps this reflects the view that doctors, whether homoeopaths or not, treat patients not people. Those individuals who prefer lay homoeopaths point out that it is always possible to liaise with their orthodox GP on issues such as drugs and the proper diagnosis of symptoms.

Ultimately, of course, it is up to the individual whether their homoeopath's medical and scientific knowledge is more important than their ability to relate to clients on a natural, one-to-one basis. It is also worth pointing out that many homoeopaths, probably the majority in fact, combine both. As always, it is best to choose a practitioner on the basis of whether they suit you personally.

Homoeopathy on the NHS Though the majority of GP homoeopaths practise privately, homoeopathy is available on the NHS at a number of specialized hospitals and out-patient clinics; simply ask your GP for a referral. Waiting times vary from about 2 months to just over a year.

Apart from cost, one of the advantages of the homoeopathic hospitals is that they offer a variety of therapies. At the Royal London Homoeopathic Hospital, therapies such as acupuncture, manipulative medicine (osteopathy/chiropractic), nutritional therapy and relaxation training are offered alongside homoeopathy. Physiotherapy and occupational therapy are also available. In theory, an individual could go for a homoeopathic treatment, have manipulation to improve mobility and learn some physiotherapy exercises to maintain any improvements.

The down side is that this might not be quite how it works in practice and that homoeopathic physicians working in a hospital setting might be too pressured for time to give proper homoeopathic consultations. It can also be hard to build up a relationship with a hospital doctor. Finally of course, you might live too far from a homoeopathic hospital to make regular visits feasible.

Homoeopathy: a Summary

- Homoeopaths use small doses of common substances in pill form to treat disease.

- Homoeopathy appears to be particularly effective in the treatment of secondary symptoms, especially recurrent infections such as 'glue ear'.
- Some homoeopaths say that they are able to treat learning disability and behaviour problems, though there is some disagreement about this.
- Homoeopathy appears to be free of side-effects.

Resources

For the location of your nearest medically qualified homoeopath, send an SAE to:

The British Homoeopathic Association
27a Devonshire Street
London W1
Tel: 071 935 2163

To find a registered lay homoeopath, send an SAE to:

The Secretary
The Society of Homoeopaths
2 Artizan Road
Northampton NN1 4HU
Tel: 0604 21400

For a referral to a homoeopathic hospital or clinic, simply ask your GP. Hospitals are located in Bristol, Glasgow, London and Tunbridge Wells with out-patient clinics at Liverpool, Manchester and Northwich (Mid-Cheshire).

HERBAL MEDICINE

Introduction to Herbal Medicine

Herbs have been used for healing for many thousands of years, in fact many modern drugs are based on original herbal remedies. Perhaps the most well known of these is aspirin, which contains a substance similar to that found in the bark of willow trees. Herbalists believe that by producing medicine directly from plants, they can provide a remedy that is safer, gentler and more effective than an equivalent drug.

There are a number of different systems of herbal medicine. Most cultures have developed their own characteristic form of herbalism and in some, elaborate systems of diagnosis and treatment have evolved. Typically, herbs are ascribed certain qualities, for example, cool, bitter or stimulating, and used according to the deficiencies or excesses of those qualities in the patient: disease states believed to result from heat are treated with 'cooling' herbs; those from languor with 'stimulating' herbs and so on.

Chinese herbal medicine is a particularly interesting example of traditional herbalism. Practitioners of Chinese medicine believe that our health is determined by the flow of a vital force or energy called *chi*. This *chi* must flow in the correct strength and quality through the body for health to be maintained. Just as an acupuncturist will use needles to correct energy imbalances, so a herbalist will prescribe herbs. A number of traditional Chinese remedies have been shown to be effective by scientific trial: in one recent study, a herbal preparation was found to be of benefit for certain sub-groups of people with eczema.

Modern medical herbalism tends to place less emphasis on the 'traditional' qualities of herbs. Herbalists are taught the medical actions and uses of different herbs in terms of their chemical constituents and they prescribe accordingly. However, this is not a simple case of 'one disease, one herb'. Medical herbalists take complex information about various systems of the body and build up a picture that will be different for each client they see, even for those with similar medical conditions.

Herbalists claim that the medicine they practise is much safer than drug therapy. They point out that whereas drugs based on herbal cures contain only one 'active in-

gredient', herbs contain many substances and so any
potential toxic effect is buffered. For example, whereas the
use of aspirin can lead to stomach problems, the use of
willow bark rarely leads to such complications, in fact,
herbalists sometimes use willow bark to *treat* stomach
symptoms.

Though many orthodox doctors have reservations about
the way in which herbal medicine is practised – some
point out that boiling up a herb in water is unlikely to give
a precise dose – many are willing to accept that herbal
remedies can have beneficial effects on health.

Visiting a Practitioner

The first visit to a herbal practitioner is generally the longest.
The herbalist will take an extensive case history by asking
a variety of questions regarding symptoms, diet, lifestyle
and the functioning of the various systems of the body,
even those that might appear to be unrelated to the problems at hand. Traditional herbalists may also use techniques such as pulse diagnosis. The aim is to gain an
overall picture so that the 'root cause' of ill-health can be
established.

To give an example, it is known that certain herbs contain substances which have anti-inflammatory effects.
However, these herbs are not prescribed indiscriminately
to everyone with arthritis. A herbalist is much more likely
to take a more elliptical approach, perhaps noticing and
treating problems of elimination such as constipation or
insufficient sweating. Practitioners say that joint symptoms often improve if such treatment is successful.

Herbs can be used in a variety of different forms. In
health stores, you will often find capsules containing dried
herbs. However, few herbalists use such preparations:
most use ready-made syrups (where the herb has been
boiled in water, with sugar added as a preservative) or
tinctures (where alcohol has been used) but it is not un-

common for practitioners to make up preparations themselves, sometimes even picking the herbs fresh from the garden. Herbs can also be used in ointments and poultices.

Herbal preparations sometimes smell unpleasant, but not unbearably so and there is often an invigorating or tonic effect after taking a dose. A problem that some parents experience is that children will sometimes refuse to take herbal medicine because of its taste. This problem is exacerbated by the fact that herbal remedies need to be taken in relatively large quantities, for example, as a cup of tea. Whereas it is generally possible to get a uncooperative child to take a pill, getting them to drink a whole cup of unpleasant tasting tea is a different thing altogether.

Herbs are generally slow to act so practitioners are usually in no hurry to change treatment if results are initially unimpressive. However, if you are worried about the pace of progress, do discuss this with your herbalist.

Herbal Medicine Treatment

Herbal medicine is often used in a similar way to homoeopathy. For example, practitioners of both therapies say that, though they can often treat arthritis or skin conditions, their work is less appropriate for problems such as low back pain or stroke. It is therefore not surprising that the main use of herbal medicine for people with cerebral palsy and allied conditions is, like that of homoeopathy, the treatment of secondary symptoms, particularly those that recur.

One of the benefits of herbal medicine most commonly reported by people with disabilities appears to be an improvement in the systems of digestion and elimination. Many herbalists are confident of their ability to control symptoms such as indigestion, vomiting, constipation or irritable bowel syndrome and this confidence appears to be justified by the experience of clients.

A herbalist who has worked with disabled people says

that her clients often experience problems with digestion. This is because movement of the body – walking, standing up, twisting – encourages movement in the intestines. So if an individual's mobility is restricted, if they spend much time sitting or lying down, it is likely that their digestive system will not work efficiently. Such problems can be exacerbated by spasticity in the stomach muscles. The herbalist has used a variety of different herbal remedies to treat digestive problems in adults and children, and she claims that she often has successful results.

There is some scientific support for these claims. Trials have shown that ginger is effective against nausea and vomiting, and that peppermint oil can be helpful for irritable bowel syndrome. However, it would be a mistake to restrict herbs to the role of 'digestive tonics'. Modern medicines based on herbal remedies have actions as diverse as increasing urine production, preventing malaria and treating heart disease, and herbalists do aim to treat the full range of symptoms.

Considerable attention has recently been focused on Chinese herbalism for eczema. As pointed out above, one particular remedy has been shown to be beneficial by a well-controlled scientific trial. As yet, it is unclear whether this type of remedy is successful for eczema related to disabilities, for example, Down's syndrome.

Herbal Medicine and Infection

Another area in which herbalists are reputed to have had considerable success is in the treatment of recurrent infections:

> The herbs have been wonderful for Sylvia's chest infections: she very rarely gets colds or flu nowadays.

It is useful to draw a comparison between herbal medicine and aromatherapy. The oils used in aromatherapy are extracted from plants and so it is not surprising that there are similarities between the two therapies. Earlier in this chapter (page 67) the effects of aromatherapy on recurrent infections were discussed. It was pointed out that not only were there anecdotal reports of benefit but also that there is actually some scientific evidence that demonstrates that aromatherapy oils are effective against bacteria and other microbes.

The following general points about the treatment of recurrent infection apply equally to herbal medicine and aromatherapy:

1. A course of treatment may reduce the frequency of infections.
2. Remedies can be kept at home to be used 'as needed', for whenever an infection recurs.
3. Infections that appear to be susceptible to treatment include respiratory infections, such as colds and flu, urinary tract infections, such as cystitis, and skin infections, such as those involved in some forms of acne.
4. One of the advantages of complementary medicine in the treatment of recurrent infections is freedom from unwanted side-effects. That said, no herb or oil should be over-used.
5. As always, complementary medicine should not be seen to replace orthodox treatment. Herbs should not be used *instead* of antibiotics prescribed by a doctor. If treatment is successful, it may be possible to avoid repeat prescriptions of antibiotics.

Herbal Medicine for Sleeplessness and Irritability

Aromatherapy and herbalism are also similar in that they can be used to calm and soothe. A number of herbs, like essential oils, are said to have sedative properties; some, for example, valerian and lavender, have been shown to be effective by well-controlled scientific trials. A number of people have found that herbs prescribed in the form of teas are particularly helpful. In addition to aiding sleep, sedative herbs have been used to soothe distracted and irritable children. One intriguing possibility is that this might reduce frequency of epileptic seizures in affected individuals. Though there has been some research in China that suggested that this might be the case, it is not really known whether herbal medicine could be of benefit in epilepsy.

One final point worth making is that, for many of those who try herbalism, one of the most marked effects can be a feeling of general well-being. This can be true even when distressing symptoms have not been helped:

> You know, though the herbs haven't done much for my painful feet, they've made me feel so well in myself. I feel on top of the world!

Herbal Medicine in Practice

In the UK, practitioners of modern herbal medicine are represented by the National Institute of Medical Herbalism: registration follows a 4-year course of training, a period of clinical practice and an examination. Members use the letters MNIMH; fellows use FNIMH.

Chinese Herbalism The Council for Acupuncture is an affiliation of five separate organizations. If you are primarily interested in herbalism, you can either contact the Council stating your wishes, or you can contact the appropriate member organizations direct. These are the International Register of Oriental Medicine (UK), the Register of Traditional Chinese Medicine and the Chung San Acupuncture Society.

Herbal medicine is also available over the counter at health stores. Self-help herbalism is unlikely to be as effective as a professional consultation: in fact, many herbalists think that the health store remedies are a travesty of true herbal medicine. See Chapter 5 for further information.

Herbal Medicine: a Summary

- Herbal medicine is the use of plants and plant extracts to treat disease.
- Herbal medicine has been reported to be of benefit for indigestion, constipation and diarrhoea.
- Practitioners of herbal medicine have also claimed to have some success in the treatment of recurrent infections in disabled people.
- Some herbs are gentle sedatives and have been used to soothe irritable children and promote sleep.

Resources

National Institute of Medical Herbalism
41, Hatherly Road
Winchester
Hants

Council for Acupuncture
179 Gloucester Place
London NW1 6DX

International Register of Oriental Medicine (UK)
4 The Manor House
Colley Lane
Reigate
Surrey RH2 9JW

Register of Traditional Chinese Medicine
19 Trinity Road
London N2 8JJ

Chung San Acupuncture Society
15 Porchester Gardens
London W2 4DB

NUTRITION

Introduction to Nutrition

There are few subjects in medicine that cause as much controversy and disagreement as that of nutrition. At one extreme, many orthodox physicians play down the idea that diet could play a role in any more than a very few conditions. At the other, there are numerous unqualified cranks and faddists who claim that their particular diet is the one true way to health, and a cure for many diseases.

Disability complicates matters even further. Few authorities on nutrition pay much attention to the needs of disabled people, who may, for example, need to eat less than able-bodied individuals. In cerebral palsy, the use of a wheelchair, and problems with spasticity, may interfere with appetite and digestion. Feeding problems may create additional complications in some cases.

There are three aspects of nutrition that are worth considering in cerebral palsy and related conditions: basic nutrition, food sensitivity and the use of nutritional supplements.

Basic Nutrition

Human beings require nutrients such as fats, proteins, minerals and vitamins. They also require energy, such as that found in sugars and starch. If a person obtains an insufficient quantity of a nutrient, a specific deficiency disease may result. For example, if a child does not receive enough vitamin B1 through the diet, he or she will develop beri-beri, a condition that affects the nerves and muscles. Disease is also associated with excess of foods. Over-eating has been linked to a number of conditions including heart disease, stroke, cancer and diabetes.

Though overt deficiency diseases are rare in the West, there are a number of reasons why they may affect disabled people. People who use wheelchairs, for example, often have low appetites; moreover, problems with money, transport and access can lead to a reliance on convenience foods and restrict the consumption of fresh fruit and vegetables. Some adults who have cerebral palsy may also have problems in preparing fresh food. This has led some authorities to suggest that disabled people should consider supplementing their diet with a general multivitamin and mineral pill as a precautionary measure against deficiency disease.

Although not strictly a deficiency, lack of fibre in the diet can lead to a number of health problems, the most notable of which is constipation. This appears to be such a common condition in cerebral palsy and other disabilities that an increase in the amount of fibre in the diet has been widely recommended. However, many foods that are high in fibre, wholemeal bread for example, are rather bulky and difficult to chew and this can cause problems for some people. One suggestion is to liquidize fibre-containing foods; more orthodox remedies include bulking agents that can be taken in pill form.

Food Sensitivity

Surprising as it may sound, certain everyday foods can cause illness in susceptible individuals. This is called food sensitivity, a term that encompasses two very separate (though often confused) concepts: food allergy and food intolerance.

Some people are allergic to particular foods in the same way that others are allergic to pollen, cat's hair or cleaning fluid. When they come into contact with a culprit food, they get a reaction, such as a skin rash, almost immediately. Other people have what is known as a food intolerance: this is when the reaction to an offending food is much slower, and when the symptoms that are caused are more varied than for allergy.

Another major difference is that whereas individuals with food allergy are generally aware of their condition, most people with a food intolerance do not suspect that their health problems are food related. The only way that this can be discovered, and remedied, is by trying a special diet known as an elimination diet.

There are a number of difficulties in trying to assess the importance of food intolerance for the purposes of this book. Firstly, many of the symptoms that have been linked to food intolerance are also common in conditions such as cerebral palsy. For example, food intolerance has been linked to indigestion and bowel problems. It has also been linked to hyperactivity and some cases of epilepsy. It can thus be particularly difficult for an individual or parent to know whether a certain symptom might be related to diet or is purely a result of damage to the nervous system.

Another important point is that the food intolerance diets work by restricting the number of different foods that are eaten. Many adults and children with disabilities may already have a number of problems with their diet: there may be difficulties in feeding or in preparing food and opportunities for shopping may be restricted. Some children can also be 'picky' about the food they eat:

A friend suggested this wheat-free diet for Cynthia. But what with her stomach problems and all, it's difficult enough to feed her as it is. I don't know what she would take if we cut out bread.

It would perhaps not be even worth mentioning food intolerance diets if it were not for the fact that many parents have found one particular diet so useful for one particular set of symptoms:

The recurrent infections cleared up within a week of cutting out milk products.

The homoeopath suggested a milk-free diet and that has helped enormously with the constant catarrh. The eczema has also improved.

The milk-free diet includes cutting out milk, cheese, butter and all other milk products. Suitable sources of energy, B vitamins and calcium need to be substituted, and this is one of the reasons why it may be advisable to experiment with this diet only in consultation with a trained practitioner (see below).

Nutritional Supplementation

The taking of nutritional supplements such as vitamin and mineral pills is a particularly controversial subject. Some people are pressing the government to restrict the availability of vitamin and mineral supplements; others advocate that large doses of supplements should be taken routinely, even by those who are fit and well.

There are a number of observations worth making. Firstly, there are a number of reasons why disabled people might be advised to take some general multivitamin and mineral supplement (see above). Secondly, though the use of high doses of vitamins has been promoted as a 'cure' for various conditions, including Down's syndrome and learning disability, scientific studies have failed to show that this 'megadose' therapy has benefit. Moreover, side-effects from this type of therapy are not uncommon.

Two subjects worthy of particular attention are essential fatty acids and the use of individually tailored nutritional supplementation:

1. *Essential fatty acids* are similar to vitamins in that they are substances that play a vital role in human metabolism and must be taken into the body in the form of food. They can be found in linseeds, vegetable oils, liver and fish. However, their activity is blocked by what are known as 'saturated fats', which are found in fatty meat, cheese and butter.

   Increasing the amount of essential fatty acids available to the body can be achieved by boosting the intake of foods such as oily fish while reducing consumption of saturated fats, and/or by taking a supplement of evening primrose oil (EPO) or fish oil (EPA). This has been found to have been of benefit in rheumatoid arthritis, heart disease and eczema. Of special interest from the point of view of this book is that essential fatty acid supplementation has been shown to be of benefit for bowel problems such as irritable bowel syndrome and skin problems such as eczema, both of which are common in disabled adults and children.

2. *Individually tailored supplementation.* With the possible exception of autism, the use of high doses of vitamins as a cure for a specific disability does not stand up to scientific scrutiny. However, some practitioners assess and treat nutritional deficiencies on an individual basis. One of their beliefs is that some individuals might eat a perfectly healthy, balanced diet yet remain deficient in one or more essential nutrients. This is normally ascribed to defects in the body's ability to absorb and/or use certain vitamins and minerals.

One of the more controversial aspects of this form of treatment concerns how vitamin and mineral deficiencies are assessed. Some practitioners use procedures that have either been discredited (applied kinesiology), had doubt cast upon them (hair analysis) or are simply unproven and unusual (Vega testing). Others, however, are orthodox doctors who have access to standard laboratory tests, and who are able to diagnose and treat vitamin and mineral deficiencies with some degree of sophistication.

Nutrition in Practice

There are a number of complications and uncertainties about the role of nutrition in the management of cerebral palsy and allied conditions. You would therefore be wise to be cautious in your choice of practitioners and dietary regimes.

Your choice will also depend on the course of action you are considering. If you are considering using some general multivitamin and mineral, an essential fatty acid supplement such as evening primrose oil or some general dietary modification, such as increasing dietary fibre, it may not be strictly necessary to contact a professional practitioner. You might want to keep your GP informed but, apart from that, these simple measures are really a personal, rather than a professional issue.

If you wish to experiment with a food intolerance approach, such as a milk-free diet, you should consider doing this with the advice and support of a professional practitioner. At the very least, you might want to check with your GP that the diet you are considering is nutritionally adequate. Your GP might refer you to a dietician, who is a specialist similar to a physiotherapist, and who will be able to give you appropriate advice.

One problem that you might encounter is that many GPs, and surprisingly, many dieticians too, are prejudiced against the idea that food can play an important role in healthcare. More often than not, the phrase 'all-round, well-balanced diet' will be used as the be-all-and-end-all of matters. If you have decided to try a particular course of action, for example, a milk-free diet to help with catarrh and recurrent infections, stick to it: politely inform your GP or dietician that this is something that you would like to try and that their role is not to talk you out of it, but to offer guidance and support.

You may wish to contact a practitioner who specializes in dietary approaches, for example, if you would like to have an individualized assessment of your, or your child's, nutritional status. In this case, there are a number of organizations that can put you in contact with an appropriately qualified practitioner. Orthodox medical doctors who are interested in diet are registered by the British Society for Nutritional Medicine and by the British Society for Allergy and Environmental Medicine.

A number of different sorts of complementary practitioners may give advice on diet. Naturopaths rely heavily on nutritional supplementation and dietary change, though herbs, hydrotherapy and osteopathic techniques also form part of their work. Many herbalists and homoeopaths have an interest in diet. Finally, some practitioners work mainly, or exclusively, with dietary manipulation. Such practitioners may describe themselves as 'nutrition consultants', others as purveyors of 'natural health services', yet others use the label 'allergists' or 'clinical ecologists'.

Because disability represents somewhat of a special case in nutrition, you would be wise to be conservative in your choice of practitioner. The advantage of an orthodox doctor specializing in nutrition over a complementary nutritionist is simply that they are more highly trained and experienced, and thus better able to deal with a less routine case such as a person with cerebral palsy. The disadvantage of doctors who specialize in nutritional medicine is that most practise privately and, presumably, expensively. If as a result you do consider a complementary nutrition practitioner, you should liaise with your GP over their recommendations (see above).

Nutrition: a Summary

- Considerable controversy surrounds the role of diet in disease.
- It is likely that some disabled people do not receive adequate vitamins and minerals from their diet. Such individuals may wish to consider taking a general multivitamin and mineral supplement.
- It has been widely reported that certain dietary changes are beneficial for recurrent chest infections.
- The use of high dose vitamin pills as a treatment for disabilities is not supported by the scientific literature.

Resources

The two societies for doctors interested in nutritional medicine are:

British Society for Nutritional Medicine
Stone House
9 Weymouth Street
London W1N 3FF
Tel: 071 436 8532

British Society for Allergy and Environmental Medicine
'Acorns'
Runsey Road
Cadnam
Southampton SO4 2NN
Tel: 0703 812124

To obtain a consultation with a dietician, ask your GP for a referral.
Organizations of complementary practitioners of nutrition:

British College of Naturopathy and Osteopathy
6 Netherhall Gardens
London NW3 5RR
Tel: 071 435 6464

Nutrition Consultants' Association
51 Robinson Meadow
Ledbury
Herts HR8 1SX
Tel: 0531 5934

The Society for the Promotion of Nutritional Therapy
2 Hampden Lodge
Hailsham Road
Heathfield
East Sussex TN21 8AE
Tel: 0435 867007

Send £1 for a list of members in your area.

OTHER THERAPIES

There are a number of techniques which, though some-times classed as complementary medicine, fall outside the scope of this book. A short description of each is given below. The resources section at the end of the section contains information and advice on finding suitable practi-tioners.

COUNSELLING

Everyone experiences emotional difficulties at some point in their life and at such times it can be valuable to talk things over with someone. There are some occasions when it might be most helpful if that person were a pro-fessional counsellor.

The term 'psychotherapy' is often used in addition to, or in place of, the term 'counselling'. Some people use coun-selling to refer to the provision of short-term emotional support, whereas psychotherapy is seen as going some-what deeper, exploring unconscious issues and long-term trends. However, the two terms are seen as synonymous for the purposes of this section.

There are two major misconceptions about counselling. Firstly, most people associate counselling with 'head shrinks', typically white-haired men with bow ties, thick European accents and a tendency to talk about sex. In fact, most modern counselling is more like a serious chat with a wise friend or teacher. Secondly, it is commonly believed that you have to be 'wrong in the head' to need counsel-ling. Consequently, many people avoid counselling be-cause they don't want to see themselves in such a light. The fact is that perfectly normal, sane people do encounter emotional difficulties and that many have been enabled to lead fuller and more contented lives through counselling.

There is increasing acknowledgement that counselling can help deal with the emotional difficulties that sometimes result from being disabled or having a disabled child. A recent innovation is what is known as 'peer counselling'. This is when counsellors for disabled people are disabled themselves. The resources listing below has information about peer counselling.

Counselling provides an opportunity to identify problems and explore feelings. For example, during a counselling session, a person might be able to discuss fears and worries about actions they have taken in the past. Talking about a fear or worry often goes some way towards alleviating it.

There are many different forms of counselling. This can be confusing for people who are worried about choosing the right sort of counselling. Fortunately, most counsellors learn a variety of techniques and use whichever is appropriate for the client. The most important consideration in deciding on counselling is choosing the right practitioner, rather than choosing the right particular form of therapy. A counsellor will often set up an interview with a prospective client before starting any counselling sessions. This gives the client an opportunity to judge whether they feel that a particular practitioner could be of help to them.

Finally, it is worth pointing out that counselling need not necessarily be a long-term project. Sometimes just one or two sessions can be helpful, perhaps in the case of some immediate crisis. Telephone help-lines can be particularly helpful in this respect.

Resources

Most counselling takes place in private settings or by the use of a telephone helpline.

For private counsellors in your area:

British Association for Counselling
37a Sheep Street
Rugby
Warwicks CV21 3BY
Tel: 0788 578328

Specialist services:

CARE
Arlington Park House
Sutton Lane
London W4 4HD
Tel: 081 994 0578
Counselling centre specializing in disability and long-term illness.

Derbyshire Centre for Integrated Living
Long Close
Cemetery Lane
Ripley
Derbyshire DE5 3HY
Tel: 0773 742165
Specialist peer counselling services available.

Cerebral Palsy Helpline
Tel: 0800 626216
Telephone helpline

The Association to Aid the Sexual and Personal Relationships of People with a Disability
286 Camden Road
London N7 0BJ
Tel: 071 607 8851
Provides appropriate leaflets and operates a telephone counselling service.

RELATE Marriage Guidance
Herbert Gray College
Little Church Street
Rugby CV21 3AP
Tel: 0788 573241

The Samaritans
Check your phone book for your local group's number.
24-hour telephone helpline, but specialist counselling is
not available.

HYPNOTHERAPY

Hypnotherapy can be thought of as a technique to master
the power of the mind. It is a two-stage process. First, an
intense state of relaxation is induced. This is known as a
trance. Secondly, suggestions are given to bring about a
healing effect. For example, the suggestion that 'my hand
feels cool and free of pain' can be used for pain relief.

Like counselling, hypnotherapy suffers from several
popular misconceptions. Firstly, hypnotism isn't about
falling into the power of a charismatic (and potentially
evil) other. Even when induced by a therapist, all hypnosis is
essentially self-hypnosis: it is about self-control, not control by someone else. Secondly, being hypnotized is not
some form of occult state brought on by strange and unknown means. It is quite possible to fall into a trance quite
naturally during everyday life (for example, during a deep
reverie). Moreover, the suggestions in hypnotherapy are
similar to those that you or I might use as a commonplace:
for example, telling someone they 'look great' has a
markedly different effect to asking them whether they are
ill.

There has been little writing or research on hypnotherapy
for conditions such as cerebral palsy. Certainly hypnosis
can be an excellent way of inducing deep relaxation, the
benefits of which are discussed on page 115. For instance,
after a course of hypnotherapy, one father noticed in his
daughter:

> Less tension, a wry smile where tears and temper tantrums
> would have been the order of the day, confidence to have a go
> and ask questions, gradual (and now complete) cessation of
> the night frights.

Less is known about the use of hypnotherapy specifically for affecting mobility and muscle function in disabled people.

Resources

Though group and individual hypnotherapy is sometimes available in hospital settings, most practice takes place privately. A number of authorities have advised consulting a doctor hypnotherapist, rather than a non-medical counterpart. One of the reasons given is that there is a particularly large number of training institutions and registering bodies and that standards vary widely.

For medically qualified hypnotherapists contact:

British Society of Medical and Dental Hypnosis
42 Links Road
Ashtead
Surrey KT21 2HJ
Tel: 0372 273522

For 'lay' hypnotherapists try:

National College for Hypnotherapy and Psychotherapy
12 Cross Street
Nelson
Lancs

UK College of Hypnotherapy and Counselling
10 Alexander Street
London W2 5NT
Tel: 071 727 2006

ART THERAPY

Art therapies divide along the traditional distinctions between different artistic forms. There is music therapy, dance therapy, drama therapy and art therapy itself, which, when used in a specific sense, refers to painting, collage and sculpture.

In work with people with learning disabilities, artistic therapies can be used as a medium of learning and social interaction. For example, banging on a drum as a music therapist plays the piano can be an excellent way of developing communication skills. Art therapies can also provide stimulation in the form of different sounds, colours and textures. Moreover, they can sometimes be helpful for physical development: music therapy can help develop a sense of rhythm and art therapy can improve control of the hands.

Some practitioners, however, see art therapies in much more simple terms: creativity is healthy, and whether somebody sings, draws or dances, the act of expression will itself be health promoting.

Resources

Art therapies are often available at special schools, units and hospitals. Some practitioners are also available for private work.

The British Society for Music Therapy
69 Avonlea Avenue
East Barnet
Herts EN4 8NB

The Nordoff Robbins Music Therapy Centre
3 Leighton Place
London NW5 2QL
Tel: 267 6296

The British Association of Art Therapy
13c Northwood Road
London N6 5LT

The British Association of Drama Therapists
PO Box 98
Kirby, Moorside
York YO6 6EX

BIOFEEDBACK

A biofeedback machine gives individuals information about their body that they would not otherwise be able to obtain. This information can then be used to help them regulate functions that are normally beyond their control. For example, a biofeedback device might be placed in the heel of a child's shoe. When the heel is lifted from the shoe, as would happen if the heel twisted upward and outward, an alarm would sound, reminding the child that he or she is adopting a position likely to complicate mobility problems. Over the course of time, the child will learn to keep the feet in the best position for standing and walking, and, after a while they will be able to do this without having to be hooked up to the measuring instruments.

The use of biofeedback machines by physiotherapists is increasing, especially in the USA. In disability work, they have been used to regulate continence, decrease spasm, control muscular tension and, as in the example above, promote correct posture and walking.

Biofeedback is a complex technique that uses high-technology and requires considerable medical expertise. As such, it would be wise to avoid practitioners of biofeedback who are not medically trained.

Resources

Though some physiotherapists do make use of biofeedback, it is rarely available on request.

UNORTHODOX TECHNIQUES

The difference between complementary medicine, such as acupuncture, and unorthodox techniques, such as Conductive Education, is explained on pages 2–5. Some well-known unorthodox techniques are described below. They are generally aimed at children and seek to improve the main symptoms of disability.

CONDUCTIVE EDUCATION

The principle of conductive education is that disorders of movement, such as those associated with cerebral palsy, are actually a form of learning difficulty. Rather than being a method of 'treatment' (such as physiotherapy or surgery), conductive education concentrates on teaching. Children go through a series of movements under the guidance of a special teacher known as a 'conductor'. The movements are devised in such a way that they form the elements of a skill such as grasping or balance. The movements may be accompanied by a song or a rhyme, often describing the activity being undertaken. For example, in a walking programme, children might sing 'Right heel, right toe, left heel, left toe' in time to their movements.

Conductive education is a total approach that requires total commitment: rather than a one-hour session once or twice a week, conductive education typically involves five full 8-hour days a week. This is because children are taught the regular parts of an educational curriculum in addition to undertaking activities related to improving physical functioning.

Conductive education remains a controversial technique. Critics have pointed out that it is difficult to make an objective evaluation of the technique. However, it is clear that many children have had successful experiences and have improved greatly on the programme.

Conductive education, previously only available in Hungary, is becoming more widely practised in the UK. More information can be found from Scope who are developing a number of training and assessment centres.

DOMAN-DELCATO: PATTERNING

Patterning is one of a number of therapies that are based on the theory that if a child's brain has been damaged (for example, in cerebral palsy), it may be 'reprogrammed' by stimulating the child in a special way. Developmentalists (proponents of patterning) believe that this encourages functioning parts of the brain to take over the jobs of the areas that have been destroyed.

The basic principle of patterning is that each stage of a child's development prompts subsequent stages by stimulating the brain. Crawling, for example, causes a particular set of nerves to fire and it is believed that this allows the brain to grow and develop in order to control the more complicated movements involved in walking.

Patterning therapy consists of sets of exercises designed to overcome blocks in development. For example, the *cross pattern* exercise mimics the action of crawling: the child lies on his or her back, with one person either side moving the limbs back and forth, and one turning the head to the left and right.

Like conductive education, patterning is very time and labour intensive: some institutes recommend up to 8 hours a day of exercise, though 2 or 3 hours is more common. Because this exercise is carried out at home, and because patterning often requires two or three people per child, a family must recruit a number of volunteers to help with the programme. This requires considerable dedication on the part of the family, especially as institutes of patterning recommend that the therapy must be continued for up to 2 years before it is possible to decide whether or not it is being effective.

Doman-Delcato is a controversial therapy, and there is conflicting evidence as to its success. Some people are critical of the huge investment of time and energy that is required of parents: others say that patterning helps families participate in the care of a child.

There are also grounds for complaint in the way in

which developmentalists present information to parents. Booklets about patterning are crammed full of miraculous case histories ('Though pronounced deaf 2 years ago, John can not only hear sounds but understand some spoken words, after only 5 months on our programme'). Developmentalists also tend to frame the debate so that those in favour of patterning are seen as the champion of the child ('We believe in your child, we're not frightened of "impossible" objectives!') whereas those who raise even the mildest query or doubt are pictured as jaundiced cynics, defeatists bent on crushing hope and untapped potential. Needless to say, this tends to prevent informed debate on the subject. See the Resources section for contact organizations for patterning.

HOLDING THERAPY

Holding therapy developed in the United States as a specific treatment for autism. Dr Martha Welch, the creator of the therapy, believes that the attachment between parent and child is of central importance in autism. In particular, the parent can help overcome the fear and insecurity that may underlie the behaviour of autistic children.

Holding therapy takes the form of sessions of hugging and holding, in which the parent insists on comforting the child, even if the child resists this. However, holding is not a self-help technique. The involvement of a professional is normally required, not only because the holding itself must be conducted sensitively but also because it often proves emotionally difficult for the parent. In such cases, the parent may well need the support and advice of a professional.

Holding therapy might be easy to criticize: it seems invasive and cruel, and certainly the claim that it is a 'cure' for autism should not be taken on trust. However, there are orthodox medical practitioners who believe that holding therapy can play an important role as part of a combination of treatments designed to improve security and communication.

BOBATH

Bobath is used by so many orthodox physiotherapists, in such a wide variety of settings, that its inclusion alongside therapies such as Doman-Delcato might be seen to be inappropriate. Yet Bobath is still widely perceived to be some sort of special and unusual technique and it is on that basis that it is mentioned here.

The principle of Bobath technique is that handling a child in a special way can help inhibit abnormal movements and postures and promote effective movement. For example, a child may be placed in a sitting position on a large beach ball so that the hips and legs must be used to maintain balance. This particular regime would be used where a child tended to rely on the arms for movement while letting the legs go stiff.

In addition to working directly with children, Bobath therapists also spend much of their time teaching parents how to handle their child. As one put it: 'How a parent holds, baths and dresses a child is all part of the treatment.' Many parents welcome the chance to take an active role in the treatment of their child in such an everyday manner.

Though Bobath is widely practised in conventional settings, there is a special centre in London that provides specialist facilities and training for therapists. The address is given below.

Resources

Information and advice on conductive education is available through Scope (see page 179).

Organizations for Doman Delcato and Patterning:

The Kerland Clinic
March Lane
Huntworth Gate
Bridgewater
Somerset TA6 6LQ
Tel: 0278 429089

Centre for Brain Injury Rehabilitation
Development
131 Main Road
Broughton
Chester CH4 0NR
Tel: 0244 532047

British Institute for Brain Damaged Children
Knowle Hall
Knowle
Bridgewater
Somerset
Tel: 0278 684060

Holding Therapy:

Dr John Richer
Consultant Clinical Psychologist
Department of Paediatrics
John Radcliffe Hospital
Oxford OX3 9DU

The Mothering Centre
8 Somerset Road
Teddington
Middlesex TW11 8RS
Tel: 081 977 2813

Bobath:

The Bobath Centre
250 East End Rd
London N2

THERAPIES TO BE WARY OF

A number of therapies other than those already mentioned in this chapter are sometimes labelled as complementary medicine. These often involve unusual practices and methods. Though some of the therapies are available in the UK, it remains one of the more remarkable features of non-conventional medicine that individuals and families will often travel many thousands of miles and incur great expense to see a practitioner. It is worth speculating whether the attraction of the 'magic cure' is enhanced if it is many thousands of miles away, rather than just around the corner.

A number of therapies have been deliberately excluded from this book. You should seriously reconsider any decision to experiment with a therapy not already mentioned in Chapter 4. You should also be particularly wary if:

1. Obtaining the therapy involves a great expenditure of time and/or money, for example, if treatment is only available abroad.
2. The therapy involves the taking of substances into the body, either by mouth or by injection. The chance of negative side-effects is generally high in such therapies. In orthodox medicine, the likely benefits of drug therapy often outweigh the costs of possible side-effects: in unconventional medicine, where the benefits are debatable, this will no longer be true.
3. Dramatic or unsubstantiated claims are made for the therapy: 'Over 90 per cent of multiple sclerosis victims return to work after treatment'.
4. Pseudoscientific language is used: 'In non-technical language ... individual cells and smaller cell unions are suspended in an isotonic body compatible solution.'
5. Facile comparisons are made with conventional therapy: 'Orthodox medicine can do nothing for these poor people, whereas ...'.

See also 'How do I avoid quacks?' (Chapter 3, page 36).

Chapter 5

How to Make the Most of It

Earlier chapters of this book have been concerned with the information you need before actually starting a course of complementary treatment. Chapter 1 introduced complementary medicine; Chapter 2 attempted to answer the question: 'What should I expect from treatment?'; Chapter 3 looked at how to make decisions about complementary medicine and Chapter 4 gave you the information needed to make those decisions. This chapter is concerned with complementary medicine once it has begun, once you have actually contacted a practitioner and are about to go for an appointment.

Encouraging Liaison Between Different Health Professionals

Many disabled people have contact with large numbers of health professionals throughout their lives. For a person with cerebral palsy, these might include, among others: GPs, consultants, surgeons, physiotherapists, occupational therapists, speech therapists, social workers, health visitors, community nurses and care workers.

This 'medical cavalcade' can cause a number of problems. A common complaint among people with disabilities is that they are often treated as just another 'case', as a medical problem rather than as a human being worthy of respect as an individual. Another grievance is that 'the right hand doesn't know what the left is doing', that there is little liaison between different professionals and that this often leads to confusing and conflicting advice being given. Many disabled people also feel 'disempowered' by health professionals, saying that rather than being allowed to play an active role in treatment, they are expected to be passive and dependent recipients of advice and therapy.

The comments of parents mirror many of these complaints. One of the most common difficulties is the feeling of being shunted around from one office to another, with no continuity or coherence in care. A recent study has highlighted many of the problems faced by parents of children with cerebral palsy. One of the study's findings is that many parents feel excluded and depersonalized by their dealings with professionals; other problems identified include conflicting advice and poor liaison between professionals.

> The system forgets the person and looks at the problem.

> Conflicting advice is given by different professionals. Nothing is done if you don't phone them and have a go at them. The system is all wrong.

> The biggest worry is the lack of liaison between the professionals themselves.

Complementary medicine generally involves contact with a health professional, be it a homoeopath, an acupuncturist or practitioner of massage. As such, using complementary medicine brings the potential danger of exacerbating problems such as poor liaison and conflicting advice, and it can often become just one more disparate element in a piecemeal programme of care.

The burden for solving these problems falls very much on the individual client or parent. Though this may sometimes prove difficult, most people find that it is ultimately very rewarding. Taking charge of healthcare, coming to feel that it is you that is controlling the process and it is you who is making the decisions, can be an empowering and liberating experience.

You do not have to be an expert to take responsibility for healthcare. Many people seem to think that because health and medicine involve special knowledge, decisions should be left to professionals, after all 'Doctor knows best'. This need not be the case. To use a simple analogy: the British law is extremely complicated and there are various types of professionals trained to understand it. However, few people ask their lawyer to decide for them which type of mortgage contract to sign, or which type of will to use. Most people ask a solicitor or lawyer for advice and then choose for themselves.

Advice on Dealing with Health Professionals

Many people find that it is not always easy to say what you feel and what you need when confronted by a health practitioner, be they an osteopath or a consultant:

> It's difficult to be assertive. He's the expert and he lets you know it.

> I don't tell my GP about the homoeopathy because I fear a negative reaction.

> The people at the osteopathic clinic seem to know what they are doing and I don't want to feel that I am getting in the way.

There are many reasons why it is important to try to break through such difficulties and every individual finds his or her own way of doing so. One of the most basic techniques is to keep reminding yourself that it is you, or your child's, health that is in question and so it is you who should be making the decisions about it. Professionals are there to serve the individual, not the other way round.

However, you should try to avoid confrontations. In particular, most professionals react badly to having their professional ability questioned. This is perhaps one of the reasons why people sometimes encounter negative reactions when they mention to their doctor that they are seeing a complementary practitioner: it can seem to suggest that the doctor has failed in some way and that his or her efforts and competence have been insufficient; if the therapy being used is unusual, such as acupuncture, the doctor may even take it that they are going about such things in completely the wrong way.

It is important that you do not play on such fears. For example, when you are first raising the issue of complementary medicine, you may wish to point out that you are using it in addition to, rather than in place of, conventional therapy, and that the reason for your interest is not so much that your doctor has failed in some way, but that you would like to utilize some of the other resources on offer. It can be wise to raise issues as questions ('I was thinking of trying homoeopathy for the chest infections, what is your opinion? Can you recommend anybody?') as opposed to assertions ('I'm sick of all these antibiotics, I want to try homoeopathy.').

Another useful tip is to take a friend or relative along. This is not just because it is twice as difficult to boss two people around as it is to boss just one: a friend can offer an independent perspective and is less likely to be categorized by the health professional as just another neurotic mother or annoying patient.

This links in with perhaps the most important point about dealing with health professionals. As one mother put it:

> Act as if you are on the conveyor belt and you'll get treated as if you are on the conveyor belt.

This mother had questioned her GP about her child's need for anti-epileptic medication. Though the GP was reluctant to make any changes, the mother was persistent and, after some discussion, he consented to an attempt to wean the child off the drugs. As it turned out, the frequency of seizures increased and the child was returned to the original dose. However, the mother did not feel that the exercise had been a waste of time, or somehow proof that 'Doctor always knows best':

Because I raised the issue, and because I was able to deal with it in an intelligent and assertive way, my GP now treats me as someone who is able to make decisions for herself. I feel he respects me more and that he involves me in treatment.

Why Liaise?

There are a number of reasons why it is a good idea to ensure good liaison between your complementary practitioners and their orthodox counterparts. One of the most general points is that your GP holds some responsibility for you, or your child's, healthcare so it is important to keep him or her aware of your health plans. After all, if you visited a consultant at the hospital or went for a test, your GP would keep a record of this.

It is a good idea to ensure that a similar thing happens if you visit a complementary practitioner. For example, when doctors prescribe a new regime of drugs, they will want to see how the patient responds so that they can decide if the regime should be continued or whether any modifications should be made. Obviously, doctors are only able to make such assessments if they are aware of all the other factors that may be affecting a patient's health. An associated issue is that a course of complementary therapy often results in a reduced need for prescribed drugs. Though reducing drug intake is generally a very good idea, it is something that has to be done carefully. For example, sudden withdrawal of steroid or anti-epileptic medication can cause serious side-effects. If you foresee the possibility of altering a drug regime as a result of complementary therapy, you will need to liaise with your GP to discuss how this should be done.

There is also the point that it is much easier to keep up a good relationship with your GP if you are open and honest about your healthcare plans than if you sneak off to the osteopath in secret: such things are bound to come out at some point, and it can be embarrassing to have to explain to a doctor why you had concealed information before.

One common worry is: 'What if my doctor thinks I am a crank?' This reflects the public perception of doctors as somehow very 'anti' complementary medicine. A number of surveys cast an interesting light on this question. A 1986 study found that 38 per cent of practising GPs had received additional training in complementary medicine and that 76 per cent referred patients to colleagues who practised complementary therapy. A more recent survey has found that over 90 per cent of trainee GPs aim eventually to learn and use a complementary technique. Such interest and confidence has gone unrecognized by the public and bodes well for anyone hoping to create effective liaison between different forms of health practitioner.

The final reason to liaise is the ideal of promoting *co-working* between different health professionals. Simply speaking, this means that different professionals work together on an individual's care, each offering his or her own specialist skills as appropriate. To give a simple example: a young child with cerebral palsy has problems with seizures, spasticity and recurrent respiratory infections. The professionals involved are a GP, a consultant, a physiotherapist and an aromatherapist. The GP and consultant decide on an appropriate form of anti-epileptic medication. Though this is found to be effective, the GP is worried about repeat prescriptions of antibiotics for the colds and suggests that the parents talk to the aromatherapist about using essential oils for this purpose; the GP also asks for details of the oils used so that she can keep a record. Meanwhile, the physiotherapist and aromatherapist get in contact to discuss how their different approaches could best be combined to help the child's muscle tone and function.

Such co-operation and liaison is all too rare in practice. Though much of the blame can be placed on the way in which medicine is currently organized, for example, having different professionals situated in different areas of town, part of the responsibility for improving liaison must lie with health practitioners themselves: there have been calls for practitioners of all disciplines to resolve problems such as power conflicts and differences in language and outlook and to learn to work together.

How to Liaise

Given that, left to themselves, practitioners do not generally liaise in the most effective manner, it is usually up to the individual to make sure that this communication process does take place. Listed below are a number of suggestions of effective ways of encouraging health professionals to co-ordinate their activities:

1. Be open and honest with health professionals. Tell them exactly who you are in contact with and what they have said and done.
2. Make a list of the names, addresses and phone numbers of your practitioners and give a copy to each.
3. Try to keep records of all your visits.
4. Discuss with each practitioner how they could best complement the skills of the others you are in contact with.
5. Ask practitioners whether they have any advice or suggestions for each other.
6. Similarly, ask each practitioner if any of the others could provide useful information of any sort.

Carrying out such suggestions, however, can be hard work. Often one professional, for example, a community nurse or health visitor, can help you achieve some of the tasks outlined above. Alternatively, you can ask your GP if he or she could be the co-ordinator for your programme of healthcare; after all, this has always been one of the guiding principles of GPs' work.

Complementary and Orthodox Practitioners: What Can Go Wrong?

Despite the fact that many orthodox and complementary practitioners enjoy a good working relationship, examples of blind prejudice do occur. For example, one man who successfully tried acupuncture was advised by his doctor to 'stick the needles back into the practitioner' next time he went for a session. On the other hand, complementary practitioners have been known to encourage people to stop exercise programmes on the grounds that 'physiotherapy is bad for you'.

A useful trick for dealing with such problems is to question the grounds for the practitioner's prejudice. Asking 'How can you be so sure?' is often helpful. In either case, explain calmly and assertively why you have made a certain choice about your healthcare and emphasize that it is your health, and your decision, that counts.

However, it is probably better to try to avoid prejudice than to have to deal with it. Any complementary practitioner who makes you feel uncomfortable about your orthodox treatment is probably not worth your time, energy and money. Similarly, a GP who consistently disagrees with the decisions you make, or who puts pressure on you to change them, should probably not remain your GP. That said, there are often a number of bureaucratic barriers to changing your orthodox health professional.

But even with the most open, honest, and unprejudiced practitioners, situations may still arise when you will be given conflicting advice. This can seem particularly difficult when it happens but it also presents an opportunity to re-affirm who is in charge and for whose benefit all this is taking place:

> My osteopath thought it would be better if Ashley stopped wearing the callipers on the grounds that they were weakening her legs and preventing her from developing her own sense of balance. The physiotherapist, of course, disagreed, and gave his own reasons. Our GP could give us no advice

one way or another so we consulted a second physio: she said that though she was generally against callipers, she thought that Ashley should wear them.

There are a number of things worth thinking about in situations such as these. Firstly, ask each practitioner closely why he or she has given the advice that they have. Secondly, try and assess whether the professional concerned is in a good position to make a judgement. Had the complementary practitioner in the story above been a herbalist (to give an example of someone unlikely to have experience in training in matters of muscle tone, posture and gait), the parent might have been wise to take his or her advice with a pinch of salt. Thirdly, think about all the possible outcomes, both good and bad, including the worst and best possible case. For example, doctors have been known to persuade people with certain illnesses not to try diets that are said to be helpful. In such instances it would be worth pointing out that, in many cases, the worst possible outcome would be an unnecessary change of diet.

By the way, you should avoid 'half-way houses'. If two practitioners suggest different things, don't nod passively to both and then, for example, only take half as many pills, or only put on the callipers every other day. If you decide to compromise, you need to ask a practitioner's advice on how this can be done.

Finally, real problems between orthodox and complementary practitioners are the exception rather than the rule. The overwhelming majority of cases involve, for example, someone taking drugs and receiving acupuncture treatment and this leaves little scope for interference or problems: throughout this book it has been stressed that the therapies mentioned are *complementary* in nature and can be used with orthodox medicine without conflict.

Your Input

One of themes of this book is that complementary medicine generally involves an active approach to healthcare: one example is the taking of responsibility for co-ordinating care, as outlined above; another is the use of self-help techniques such as meditation and yoga. There are a number of other areas in which your input can be important for the progress of healthcare.

Give Your Practitioner As Much Information As You Can

Many practitioners of complementary healthcare have limited experience of disability and it is important that you tell your practitioner as much about yourself, or your child, and the condition as possible. In this respect, it can be a good idea to jot down a list to take along with you to your appointment as it is easy to forget things once you are there. Some things worth mentioning include:

1. The basic medical facts. Some practitioners may be unaware of what exactly cerebral palsy is. You might also want to explain symptoms such as spasm or athetosis (involuntary motion). If you feel uncomfortable about doing this, you can encourage your practitioner to contact your GP.
2. Tell your practitioner about the other professionals involved in you or your child's care.
3. If you are using a therapy that involves hands on work, for example, massage or osteopathy, it is important to spell out any difficulties you or your child might have with spasm. Discuss any physical positions that cause spasm and mention parts of the body that are sensitive to touch.
4. Tell your practitioner about any 'contraindications' (see page 174).
5. A number of practitioners have had problems of 'over-

stimulating' when they have worked with some disabled people. It is always possible to create problems
by causing changes to occur too fast and a number of
disabled people have encountered difficulties because
their practitioners tried to do too much, too quickly.
Mention this to your practitioner and encourage them
to go slowly and gently at first.

Diet and Lifestyle Changes

Changes in diet and lifestyle have traditionally been associated with complementary medicine. One of the reasons
for this is the holistic outlook of many complementary
practitioners (see page 1). Another is that the classic
'nature cure' of the eighteenth and nineteenth century
involved clean living, fresh air, exercise and a moderate
diet. Most people still expect to be given advice on nutrition and lifestyle when they try a complementary therapy.

In cerebral palsy and related conditions, however, the
importance of lifestyle and diet is less clear. For example,
damage to the brain caused in infancy cannot be remedied
by an alteration to the diet. There are some dietary
changes which have been reported to be useful, and these
are summarized in Chapter 4 (page 135).

Practitioners may also prescribe changes in lifestyle and
exercise. Yoga and tai chi consist entirely of special sets of
exercise: see Chapter 4 for more details. Other practitioners may suggest movement or stretching exercises, and
relaxation and breathing exercises are also common.

The important point about diet and lifestyle changes is
that they should be *negotiated* with the practitioner. It is
not a simple case of the practitioner laying down the law
and the client either following orders ('complying') or not
('failing to comply'). The practitioner's job is to suggest
changes with which the client would be able to comply. As
a result, it is the client's job to inform the practitioner what
changes would be possible and enjoyable.

So be open and honest about any difficulties you think you might have in following a course of treatment. No matter how trivial you think a problem might be, remember that the practitioner is there to serve you, not to be obeyed and that he or she may have experience of similar problems and so might be able to suggest an appropriate solution or compromise.

Self-help

One of the main ways in which an individual or parent can make an input into healthcare is by using a self-help technique. There is little question that self-help can play an important part in healthcare. One of the advantages of self-help is that it involves people in treatment, so that they play an active role in healthcare rather than just being a passive 'recipient of therapy'. For parents used to having to let health professionals take over the care of their child and for the individual who is tired of being just a 'case', this can prove to be an empowering and liberating experience. Parents who have learned a little massage and who use it on their children at home have said that they have found it to be an enjoyable and enriching experience.

Self-help also has a number of practical benefits. It is much less of a financial burden than professional practice and does not require travel, with all the attendant difficulties of time and access. It also circumvents the problem of quackery.

That said, professional practitioners are too valuable a resource to ignore. Moreover, self-help does have its limitations: there are undoubtedly certain areas of practice that individuals should avoid engaging in without consulting a professional. See Chapter 1 for a further discussion.

It is also worth relating that at least some carers find that they do not have the energy for programmes of self-help. Having to be a part-time therapist can prove just too much on top of work, family and caring for a disabled child. It is worth bearing this in mind when you consider starting or terminating any self-help activities.

Listed below are several areas in which self-help has been found to be valuable.

Good Ideas for Self-help

1. Relaxation and meditation exercises, whether learned at a class or from a book.
2. Though yoga and tai chi generally need to be learned from an experienced teacher, they can (and should) be practised at home.
3. Simple dietary modifications, such as increasing intake of fresh fruit and vegetables and other sources of dietary fibre. Some people try simple food-intolerance diets, such as a milk-free diet, without professional advice. There is disagreement as to whether or not this is a good idea (see page 137).
4. A general multi-vitamin and mineral supplement. Fatty acid supplements can also be simple to use. The use of individual supplements, for example, a vitamin A or iron supplement, is more complicated and might best be left to a professional.
5. Homoeopathic remedies for mild symptoms. Severe and recurrent problems would best be left up to a practitioner.
6. Some practitioners may offer to teach you specific therapeutic routines (see below).

Carers as Therapists

Throughout this book it has been stressed that the effectiveness of complementary medicine often depends on long-term treatment. This is because, in many cases, the benefits of therapy are relatively short term.

The problem comes in combining this need for long-term treatment with the importance of using the services of trained health professionals (see above and page 6). Clearly expense is an important issue. Many people are also worried about becoming dependent on a practitioner.

One potential solution is for carers to learn therapeutic techniques that they can use regularly at home. However, this is something that requires considerable care. Clearly no carer will become a proficient therapist merely by reading *How to* books. On the other hand, few carers have the time or inclination to take a full 3-year training in a complementary therapy. One solution is to use a model of carer and parent involvement first pioneered in physiotherapy. Physiotherapists regularly teach parents special exercises that they can use with their children at home; parents may also receive tuition in the best way to carry, bathe and dress their child. However, the physiotherapist will still want to work directly with the child and to see the parents regularly.

The equivalent in complementary medicine is to initiate and continue appointments normally for a month or two. This helps 'kick start' treatment and also gives the practitioner an opportunity to assess the particular needs of the client. After a while, the practitioner begins to involve the parent or carer more directly in the treatment session. At first, this might take the form of careful explanation. This would then evolve into hands on work, perhaps starting with the practitioner encouraging the parent to feel with their hands for say, stiffness or spasm and moving on to the use of specific therapeutic techniques, such as stretching or work on a pressure point.

Finally, the practitioner and carer would work together on a set routine that the carer could use at home. Appointments would then continue at intervals of a month or two: these allow the practitioner to assess progress, check on the carer's technique and give 'top up' treatments. Therapies appropriate for carers to work in this way are as follows:

- *Massage and aromatherapy.* Basic massage and self-massage techniques can be learned with relative ease. The aim should be gentle relaxation rather than specific changes such as an improvement in muscle tone. Aromatherapy oils can be used at home, though it is necessary to use some care. A professional aromatherapist can give advice on the suitable use of essential oils in the home. Massage appears to have a particularly useful self-help role in the treatment of constipation (see page 65).
- *Reflexology.* Some reflexology techniques can be learned with relative ease. Commonly, practitioners diagnose a particular area of the foot that needs attention and demonstrate the method of reflexology treatment.
- *Healing.* Some practitioners encourage parents or carers to develop their healing skills. This is a particularly important part of the Metamorphic technique.
- *Shiatsu.* A practitioner can teach techniques such as simple stretches. They can also locate points that require stimulation and explain to a carer how this is done.
- *Acupuncture.* As in shiatsu, practitioners can identify points on which carers can work with their hands.

The Family

Many practitioners say that treatment is often most effective when the whole family becomes involved; some practitioners have even suggested that the family should replace the individual as the object of treatment in medicine.

There are a number of reasons traditionally given for the importance of the family in healthcare. It is often pointed out that the family constitutes an important element in a person's environment, and that environment often plays an important role in causing ill-health. Another issue is that families tend to get used to, and become organized around, an individual who is sick. Families generally resist changes to their structure, such as that which would occur if an unwell individual recovered, and this can complicate the task of healthcare.

One of the immediate problems about these ideas is that it is difficult to see how they relate to a condition such as cerebral palsy. An individual's family environment is not what causes cerebral palsy; moreover, as cerebral palsy is not a disease, it is not something that can be 'recovered' from. Perhaps worst of all, ideas about the role of the family in disease seem to blame parents. As many parents of disabled children already suffer many problems relating to guilt, this can hardly be seen as a plus.

Nevertheless, thinking about the role of the family in healthcare can often be worthwhile. In particular, there is growing agreement that if somebody needs to undergo a programme of therapy, it can be beneficial for other members of his or her family to engage in some form of health promoting activity as well. This might be a complementary therapy or discipline, but it might involve an exercise programme or even a creative hobby. It is increasingly common for say, a mother of a child with cerebral palsy to receive a massage from her child's practitioner, or for a non-disabled brother to practice yoga along with his disabled sister. One centre for disabled children that provides aromatherapy has a regular 'mother's day' in which it is the parents, rather than the children, who enjoy the benefit of a relaxing massage. In other families, people have taken up running or aerobics, or changed to a healthier eating pattern.

One of the most important reasons for this family participation in therapy is connected with the way in which many disabled people come to see themselves as 'sick', and in need of medical attention, but see the able-bodied as fit and well. This self-perception is often reinforced by the often constant round of therapy and special activity which the disabled individual has to endure. If other members of the family also use complementary therapies, a person's view of themselves as different and in need of help may be moderated.

It is also worth pointing out that the sort of stimulation that a family can provide to a disabled child can have important effects on development. One immediate problem is that having a disabled child can be tiring, stressful and emotionally draining, and people who are tired, stressed and emotionally drained are not at their best for creating a stimulating and nurturing environment. Complementary therapies can be a good way of relaxing and recharging, making sure that members of the family have the energy, calmness and emotional strength to provide a worthwhile place to be for both themselves and a disabled child. To give a simple example: a mother who puts her back out would probably be doing both herself and her child more good by asking the osteopath to work on her, rather than her child.

An associated issue is that other members of a family can, at some level, resent all the attention paid to a disabled person. Parents may come to feel 'I'm so exhausted I can barely walk, but look who gets the therapy.' Similarly, brothers and sisters can sometimes come to feel ignored. Such feelings of resentment commonly exacerbate the guilt felt by so many people who live in a family with a disabled person.

Finally, of course, everybody's health care is important and a worthwhile end in itself. One obvious worry is financial: disability often causes significant financial burdens and complementary therapy can be expensive (see page 51). It would be logical for a parent to worry whether they could pay for themselves as well as their child. However, it is probably better to think of the question in terms of: how many sessions intended for my child will me and my partner take instead? In other words, it might well be wise to think of therapy for parents and family as an essential, rather than an optional extra. Your practitioner will probably be able to advise you further on this matter.

What Can Go Wrong

There are two sorts of things that can go wrong in complementary medicine. Firstly, unwanted side-effects from treatment, though rare, are not unknown. Secondly, the relationship between client or carer and the practitioner may become difficult.

Adverse Effects of Complementary Medicine

Reports of adverse side-effects from complementary medicine are rare in the medical literature; moreover, the majority do not involve the use of registered practitioners or reputable therapies. For example, an acupuncturist who caused an outbreak of hepatitis B by using unsterilized needles had previously been refused accreditation by the appropriate governing body and had been practising as an unqualified quack. Typical reports of herbal poisoning involve off-the-shelf products purchased without the advice of a practitioner. This is one of the reasons why it is advisable to consult a professional who is registered by a recognized governing body.

The most common type of side-effect from complementary therapies lasts for a few hours or days after treatment. Symptoms typically include headaches, sweating, diarrhoea, increased urination and mild muscular aches and pains. These symptoms do not normally recur, and many practitioners believe them to be a necessary stage in the healing process. Practitioners give a similar explanation for what is known as an 'aggravation reaction', which is when the symptoms of disease temporarily worsen before they improve. Therapies in which this has been reported to occur include homoeopathy, acupuncture, reflexology, cranial osteopathy, nutritional therapy and shiatsu.

Though aggravation reactions are generally harmless, they can cause complications in conditions where an exacerbation of symptoms would be dangerous. Such conditions include asthma and epilepsy, where severe, and cystic fibrosis. If you, or your child, has one of these conditions, it would be advisable to discuss the matter with your practitioner and warn them to go slowly and carefully at first.

Another side-effect of interest is that some herbal products are said to trigger epileptic seizures in sensitive individuals. This has implications for aromatherapy, as well as for herbal medicine. An effect of this type is known as a contraindication, which is when a remedy or technique should be avoided in particular cases. A list of contraindications is given below.

Contraindications of Complementary Medicine in Cerebral Palsy and Related Conditions

- Certain herbs can trigger epileptic seizures in susceptible individuals, particularly when made up into essential oils. Reputable herbalists and aromatherapists should be aware of this problem. One authority advises caution with the following oils: rosemary, sweet fennel, hyssop, sage and wormwood. This list should not, however, be seen as exhaustive.
- Yoga and tai chi must be used with caution, particularly by those with more severe disabilities. Like any form of exercise, 'pushing yourself' can lead to injuries.
- In the odd rare case, relaxation techniques can exacerbate emotional anxiety and physical tension. If this occurs, further use of the relaxation technique should not take place.
- Complementary therapies should not generally be used during acute illness, such as flu or fever. Homoeopathy and herbal medicine, and possibly acupuncture, are exceptions to this; aromatherapy can be used if massage is avoided and other methods of application employed.

- Therapies which involve touch (for example, massage, osteopathy) should avoid areas of the body affected by burns or severe skin disease.
- Care must be taken in the case of any serious disease (for example, malnutrition, malignant cancer). Though therapies can be used to relax and calm, any form of stimulation is generally to be avoided.

Difficulties in the Relationship between Practitioner and Client

Though rare, difficulties and disagreements between client and practitioner are not unknown in complementary medicine. One of the reasons why this can be especially distressing is that the client may be relying on the practitioner for help and support. The loss of trust involved in a disagreement can thus be especially hard to take.

One thing that should definitely not happen in complementary medicine is for a practitioner to wield any form of power over a client or parent. For example, the practitioner may suggest that someone makes certain changes to his or her diet, lifestyle or healthcare programme. However, it is up to the client to take or leave this advice: the practitioner should never make demands or pressure a client into a course of action.

Similarly, practitioners should never try to make a client or parent feel guilty. It is all too easy for a practitioner to blame a lack of progress on the client, either by implying that he or she is not trying or doing enough, or by referring to the role of the mind and the family in disease (see above). Even if the practitioner did have a case, it would be incumbent upon them to raise the issue without using blame and guilt.

On the other hand, there are some behaviours that parents and clients should avoid. One common problem is that of over-dependence: a number of practitioners have reported that clients have begun to call them at all times of the day and night to explain new symptoms or problems. Others have tried to extend treatment sessions beyond the agreed period. No matter how helpful, considerate and caring a practitioner might be, and no matter how wonderful the relationship you develop, health professionals are not a replacement for friends and family and you should not treat them as such.

Summary: How to Make the Most of It

- Individuals and parents can play a positive role in ensuring that healthcare leads to maximum benefit.
- Complementary medicine increases the number of health professionals working with an individual. This can sometimes exacerbate problems such as poor liaison and conflicting advice.
- It is up to the individual or parent to take control and organize an effective programme of care: encouraging different professionals to cooperate and liaise is an important part of this process.
- Individuals should remember that it is they or their child's health that is in question and that it is up to them to make the decisions.
- Self-help can be an important way of ensuring that an individual obtains maximum benefit from healthcare. This can include simple diet and lifestyle changes as well as techniques such as meditation and yoga.
- Some carers have learned simple techniques of therapies such as massage or shiatsu and found it useful to use these regularly at home.
- It can also be valuable for members of a family other than the affected individual to undertake health-promoting activities.
- It is also important to be aware of what can go wrong in complementary medicine. In particular, it is important to remain aware of what should not form part of the

relationship between a practitioner and client or parent.

- Complementary medicine has helped many people with disabilities. Making an informed choice on complementary medicine, and taking positive steps to maximise its benefit, may well help you or your child achieve better health.

Useful Addresses

OTHER USEFUL ORGANIZATIONS INCLUDING THOSE
OUTSIDE THE UK

British Organizations

Research Council for Complementary Medicine (RCCM)
60 Great Ormond Street
London WC1N 3JF
Tel: 071 833 8897
Promotes rigorous research into complementary medicine. The RCCM also runs a literature searching service for health professionals.

Council for Complementary and Alternative Medicine (CCAM)
179 Gloucester Place
London NW1 6DX
Tel: 071 724 9103
Umbrella body for acupuncture, herbal medicine homoeopathy and osteopathy. However, not all practitioners of these therapies are registered with CCAM.

Institute for Complementary Medicine
PO Box 194
London SE16 1QZ
Tel: 071 237 5165
Information on complementary medicine. Administers the British Register of complementary practitioners (see page

37) and can refer enquirers to competent therapists. Enclose a large SAE when contacting the Institute for Complementary Medicine.

The Spastics Society (to be named SCOPE
from November 1994)
12 Park Crescent
London W1N 4EQ
Tel: 071 636 5020
Britain's largest disability charity. Works and campaigns on the rights and needs of people with cerebral palsy.

SCOPE
160 Fernhead Road
London W9 3EL
SCOPE is a small charity that predates the change of name of the Spastics Society. It aims to promote the health and independence of people with severe disabilities by the use of complementary therapies.

Contact a Family
16 Strutton Ground
London SW1P 2HP
Tel: 071 222 2695
Support for families who care for children with special needs.

In Touch
10 Norman Road
Sale
Cheshire M33 3DF
Tel: 061 905 2440
Information and contacts for parents of children with special needs.

Foreign Organizations

If you have trouble locating a suitable practitioner outside the UK, try contacting one of the British organizations listed in Chapter 5.

American Academy of Osteopathy
1127 Mount Vernon Road
PO Box 750
Newark
Ohio 43058-0750
USA

Australian Council on Chiropractic and
   Osteopathic Education
941 Nepean Highway
Mornington
Victoria 3931
Australia

New Zealand Register of Osteopaths
PO Box 11 – 853
Wellington 1
New Zealand

International Society for Clinical and
   Experimental Hypnosis
PO Box 298
Belmead
New Jersey 08502
USA

American College of Nutrition
722 Robert E. Lee Drive
Wilmington
North Carolina 20927
USA

American Institute of Homoeopathy
1500 Massachusetts Avenue NW
Washington DC 20005
USA

Canadian Society of Homoeopathy
PO Box 4333
Station East, Ottawa
Canada K15 5B3

North American Society of Homoeopaths
4712 Aldrich Avenue
Minneapolis 55409
USA

Australian Institute of Homoeopathy
21 Bulah Close
Berowra Heights
Sydney NSW 2082
Australia

New Zealand Homoeopathic Society
PO Box 67095
Mt Eden
Auckland
New Zealand

New Zealand Institute of Classical Homoeopathy
24 Westhaven Drive
Tawa, Wellington
New Zealand

Australian Society of Teachers of the Alexander Technique
PO Box 529
Milsons Point
Sydney 2061
New South Wales

Canadian Society of Teachers of the Alexander Technique
460 Pamerston Boulevard
Toronto, Ontario
P7A 4A2
Canada

North American Society of Teachers of the
   Alexander Technique
PO Box 806
Ansonia Station
New York
NY 10023-0806
USA

American Association of Acupuncture and
   Oriental Medicine
National Acupuncture Headquarters
1424 16th Street NW
Suite 501
Washington DC 20036
USA

Acupuncture Ethics and Standards Organization
PO Box 84
Merrylands
NSW 2160
Australia

New Zealand Register of Acupuncturists
PO Box 9950
Wellington 1
New Zealand

National Herbalists Association of Australia
247-9 Kingsgrove Road
Kingsgrove
SA 2208
Australia

American Herb Association
Box 353
Rescue
California 96672
USA.

Further Reading

COMPLEMENTARY THERAPIES FOR DISABLED PEOPLE

Sanderson, H. and Harrison, J. with Price, S., *Aromatherapy and Massage for People with Learning Difficulties*, Hands On Publishing, 1991.

Vickers, A., *Complementary Medicine and Disability*, Chapman & Hall, 1993.

Zhao-Pu, W., *Acupressure Therapy*, Churchill-Livingstone, 1991 (aimed mainly at professionals).

SELF-HELP GUIDES

Brosnan, B., *Yoga for Handicapped People*, Human Horizons, 1986.

Catalano, E. M., *The Chronic Pain Control Workbook*, New Harbinger Publications, 1987.

Downing, G., *The Massage Book*, Penguin, 1972.

Kent, H., *Yoga for the Disabled: A Practical Self-help Guide*, Thorsons, 1985.

Long, B., *Meditation: a Foundation Course*, Barry Long Foundation, 1986.

Mitchell, L., *Simple Relaxation*, Murray, 1987.

GENERAL INTEREST

Boston Women's Health Book Collective, *The New Our Bodies, Our Selves: a Book By, For and About Women*. Penguin Books, 1989.

Most libraries stock a collection of books describing the different therapies in more detail. Though many are useful, some caution is required because many of the books are written by proponents of the therapy in question and are rather promotional in nature. Moreover, few books make mention of disability.

Index